CRYSTALS FOR BEGINNERS

The Essential Guide to the Power of Crystals for Happiness

(The Ultimate Beginners Guide to Understanding and Using Healing Crystals)

Gwendolyn Randall

Published by Harry Barnes

Gwendolyn Randall

All Rights Reserved

Crystals for Beginners: The Essential Guide to the Power of Crystals for Happiness (The Ultimate Beginners Guide to Understanding and Using Healing Crystals)

ISBN 978-1-7751430-3-1

All rights reserved. No part of this guide may be reproduced in any form without permission in writing from the publisher except in the case of brief quotations embodied in critical articles or reviews.

Legal & Disclaimer

The information contained in this book is not designed to replace or take the place of any form of medicine or professional medical advice. The information in this book has been provided for educational and entertainment purposes only.

The information contained in this book has been compiled from sources deemed reliable, and it is accurate to the best of the Author's knowledge; however, the Author cannot guarantee its accuracy and validity and cannot be held liable for any errors or omissions. Changes are periodically made to this book. You must consult your doctor or get professional medical advice before using any of the suggested remedies, techniques, or information in this book.

Upon using the information contained in this book, you agree to hold harmless the Author from and against any damages, costs, and expenses, including any legal fees potentially resulting from the application of any of the information provided by this guide. This disclaimer applies to any damages or injury caused by the use and application, whether directly or indirectly, of any advice or information presented, whether for breach of contract, tort, negligence, personal injury, criminal intent, or under any other cause of action.

You agree to accept all risks of using the information presented inside this book. You need to consult a professional medical practitioner in order to ensure you are both able and healthy enough to participate in this program.

Table of Contents

INTRODUCTION 1

CHAPTER 1: THE ESSENTIALS OF CRYSTALS AND THEIR HEALING ENERGY 3

CHAPTER 2: ALEXANDRITE 6

CHAPTER 3: UNDERSTANDING THE CHAKRAS AND THEIR CONNECTION TO CRYSTAL HEALING 29

CHAPTER 4: WHICH CRYSTALS SHOULD I USE? 65

CHAPTER 5: CRYSTALS FOR EVERYONE 78

CHAPTER 6: THE SCIENCE BEHIND CRYSTALS 89

CHAPTER 7: THE BASICS OF HEALING THROUGH CRYSTALS 99

CHAPTER 8: CRYSTAL HEALING TECHNIQUES 107

CHAPTER 9: CRYSTALS- SO PRETTY AND HELPFUL TO US 125

CHAPTER 10: ESOTERIC AND EVOLUTIONARY EXPANSION 143

CONCLUSION 188

Introduction

Thank you for choosing this book. We are about to start a journey in the fantastic world of crystal, together. I'll guide along the way, and teach you all you need to know to start using and healing with crystal.
Your life is about to get a little bit more magical. Are you ready?
Crystal healing, or as some call it, crystal energy healing, is essentially an alternative form of treatment which has been around for longer than you or I care to remember.
As with all types of holistic treatments, you get countless people who vouch for the power of crystal healing, and you get countless people who dismiss it. One of the reasons why so many people believe there's no truth in it, is because they automatically assume crystal healers believe they're able to cure serious illnesses like cancer and etc. In reality

however, this couldn'tbe any further from the truth. No reputable crystal therapist will ever make such claims. What I personally believe in, is the power of intention.

So whether your faith resides in science, physics, magic, or in none of those things, there is one thing, on which we will agree on. Where there's a will there's a way. Personally, I am convinced of this, for a straightforward reason. This theory gives me the certainty, that I and only I, am in control of my destiny, and of my possibilities. This gives me the strength to pursue my goals every day, and while I do it, I get help from my crystals. They help to set my goals, my intention and have a clear mind and a light heart.

Chapter 1: The Essentials Of Crystals And Their Healing Energy

As a novice, it is important to understand the basics of crystal before leaping into the actual process of healing. By reviewing the historical aspects of crystal healing, one can form a basic understanding of the stones' characteristics and different uses. Once you understand the general background of the practice, you can begin to explore the subject on higher levels.

The First Crystals

Nothing in life is free, especially when it is something of great importance. The high demand for crystals makes them quite expensive. Crystals are therefore, also a profitable investment where one may find true value for your money. At the beginner level, it is not recommended that one purchase an entire crystal collection, as this can be a relatively more expensive way of acquiring the stones. Your supplier and the type of crystals determine the price of your collection, and entire collections are going to cost you more either way. Therefore one should begin the spiritual journey by purchasing stones in limited quantities. The best approach is to opt for multipurpose crystals. These work as "all-rounders" and possess enough potential to carry out many tasks.

Selection Process

Selecting a healing crystal is not a simple task. You need to ensure certain qualities are present before the purchase, with special emphasis on the following tips:

The crystal should contain any cracks or chips;

Avoid falling into the common trap of choosing a stone based on its – which does not determine its true quality;

When the crystal is felt by holding it in your hand, it should provide a warm feeling, a tingle, throbbing or prickling on the skin then you may have found the perfect stone for yourself;

If you are drawn to a particular stone or have a strong feeling about it, then you should rely on your intuition and choose that stone, as feelings will play an immensely important role in determining your relation with it.

Chapter 2: Alexandrite

Alexandrite, sometimes known as 'Friday's stone' is an unusually rare stone whose scarcity is only matched by its mystery. This rarefied crystal was first discovered in Russia's Ural Mountains on the birthday of Prince Alexander the second of Russia in 1830. The first Alexandrite crystals were believed to be Emeralds due to their bright green hues. However, when the miners who found the stones viewed the stones at night by the light of the fire the stones appeared to be a brilliant red. When in the light of day the stones returned to their original deep green hues and with that a new crystal had been discovered. Alexandrite is believed to be a lucky stone that brings good fortune, joy, and love into the lives of those affected. It is a stone regularly used by skilled practitioners to boost creativity, intuition and communication skills, enhancing the abilities and creative process of the practitioner. Alexandrite activates the Crown Chakra and so has the ability to influence brain functions, the resulting energy greatly enhances psychic abilities, making astral projection possible as well as strengthening connections to higher spiritual plains and ancient knowledge. The vibrational energy emitted by Alexandrite acts to balance the psychical energy within us with that of the spiritual realm which in turn supercharges our natural abilities of transformation and manifestation giving us that extra push to truly create the life we desire. Alexandrite has been used in the healing of mental illnesses, depression and is even said to increase a man's virility. The positive effects for those suffering from head or brain-related injuries and conditions are well noted as to is Alexandrite's ability to regulate blood flow and kick-start the body's natural detoxification processes. It is a restorative stone that helps us to regain both physical and spiritual energy but ultimately, Alexandrite is a crystal that brings hope, love, and understanding to all who come into contact with it.

Colour

Green by day/Red by night (by candlelight or fire)

Birthstone

June

Zodiac

Gemini

Energetic Frequencies

Hope

Love

Healing

Balance

Chakras

The Crown Chakra

Alunite

Alunite is typically a green stone that sometimes forms with hues of red or brown and is renowned for being comprised of both yin and yang energy. The energetic frequency of this gemstone is therefore exquisitely balanced, this energy has a calming effect on anyone who comes into contact with it or on any space in which it is left for any reasonable amount of time. Alunite is a favourite stone of artists and writers due to its ability to ignite and enhance the creative process resulting in positively fascinating results. It is a crystal that stimulates motivation and strengthens concentration, which when combined with the qualities previously mentioned makes Alunite an extremely powerful stone and one that we should all regularly carry on our person. Spiritually, Alunite acts as a protective barrier surrounding us with positive energy which deflects negativity directed towards us and simultaneously boosts our levels of spiritual and mental endurance, allowing us greater levels of patience and determination in order to help us achieve personal success. It is a gemstone that wards off enemies and supports us as we strive to do the best we can, in what can sometimes be a somewhat unfair world. Alunite fortifies our ability to power on through and do the right thing no matter the circumstance which makes it the perfect crystal for those going through difficult times, are overworked or generally stretched thin. Emotionally, Alunite is perfect for suffers from exhaustion, stress, and feelings of depression, doubt, anxiety, fear, and excessive anger and frustration. Since Ancient Rome Alunite has been used in the treatment of stomach ulcers, skin irritations, and to slow down blood loss and aid coagulation and is still sold today as a cure for me who cut themselves during shaving. Alunite carries direct connections to the Sacral, Heart, and Root Chakras bringing them into proper alignment which harmonises the chakra network as a whole, grounding our body's natural vibrational field and allowing for the free movement of energy to flow throughout the body restriction free.

Colour

Green

Red/Brown

Birthstone

February

Energetic Frequencies

Healing

Protective

Calming

Creative

Chakras

The Heart Chakra

The Sacral Chakra

The Root Chakra

Amazonite

Amazonite is a much-loved stone which displays deep shades of turquoise and green and upon the first contact is believed to calm the spirit and replenish the soul. Sometimes known as 'The Stone of Truth and Courage' Amazonite empowers the individual along a journey of self-discovery leading to the discovery of one's personal truths. Its calming energy tempers wayward emotions promotes self-control and acts to release any emotional blockages or past traumas that have accumulated within the body's energetic network. Amazonite is great for cleansing and normalising the chakras; it bridges the gap between the physical body and its ethereal counterpart which dissolves inner conflict, focusses efforts and acts amplify results. Amazonite also reinforces and balances the connection between intellect (mind) and intuition (heart) creating a balanced resonance that leads to enhanced abilities and enlightenment. Reputed as carrying powerful healing properties Amazonite is believed to protect against calcium deficiency and hair loss, promotes normal brain functions and prevents infections, clears rashes and eczema, reduces symptoms relating to inflammation and increases feelings of overall wellbeing. Connection, communication and truth are brought about through Amazonite's energetic connection with the Throat Chakra and by combining this with the activating effect Amazonite can have on the Heart Chakra results in greater levels of self-worth and self-esteem. The Vibrational energy that radiates from Amazonite creates greater awareness of one's actions, one's words and the impact that we have on the people close to us. Keeping Amazonite in the home opens communication between family members reduces temper tantrums as its inner 'water-energy' guides each member of the household towards their individual goals. Amazonite is also known as a 'good luck stone' and so is a great talisman for...well...everyone. When worn as an amulet or talisman Amazonite acts a barrier to undesirable situations and people, shields the wearer from the electromagnetic radiation we are constantly exposed to and it also has the ability to absorb dangerous toxins from the environment.

Colour

Green/Turquoise

Birthstone

March

April

Zodiac

No association

Energetic Frequencies

Compassion

Healing

Love

Chakras

The Heart Chakra

The Throat Chakra

Amber

Amber has, since Neolithic times been one of the worlds most coveted treasures and not only because for its beautiful warmth of colour which is like golden honey but also because it was looked upon as a gift from the sea. The Greek word Anbar was adopted in the 14**th** century as the description of what we now call Ambergris (ambergris or grey amber) which is a solid waxy resin-like residue produced by sperm whales and is used in many of the world's most expensive perfumes and fragrances. Somewhere around the 15**th** century, the word amber was extended to include Baltic amber (yellow amber) which is fossilised sap/resin and can take millions of years to form. Amber is not technically a crystal or mineral but is still classed as an organic gemstone and is referred to in the Far East as the 'soul of the tiger'. Amber holds a strong connection with both the earth and the sun and is held in high regard for its purifying and healing properties but drawing pain and disease from the body is only the beginning for Amber, which is known to absorb, purify or purge negative and stagnant energies as well as stimulating the body's own natural healing mechanisms and processes including, regenerative and energy boosting, leaving the wearer feeling fresh and invigorated. Amber is commonly used as a protective stone for children, frequently given as a bracelet or necklace to help sooth infant teething pains or placed in a child's room to protect the room from negative outside influences. As a love gemstone Amber golden yellow or red colourings represent fertility and tenderness making it the perfect good luck talisman for increasing one's natural radiance and attracting meaningful and long-lasting love. Simply rubbing a piece of Amber unlocks its conductive energy and acts to cleanse the chakra network. Golden hues of Amber though to orange stimulate the naval or sacral chakra unblocking it and helping the wearer 'find balance' and understanding. The more yellowy hues of Amber are said to be linked to the third or solar plexus chakra allowing the wearer to freely go about their daily business without suffering the anxiety or living in fear of violating the expectations of others. Yellow Amber also aids in maintaining the body's natural flow of energy, boosting both the digestive and immune systems, boosting the wearers overall energy and warding off any feelings of fear or disappointment. When attempting to connect to information from an earlier age many spiritualists turn to Amber to help facilitate stronger connections. By passing beads made from Amber through the fingers or turning a piece if Amber in the hand when meditating it has been said that higher or expanded levels of consciousness are attainable and many shamans also claim Amber as an aid in as past life regressions.

Colour

Warm yellow/Golden honey

Red/Orange

Green

Black

Birthstone

November

Zodiac

Aquarius

Cancer

Leo

Pisces

Scorpio

Energetic frequencies

Healing

Luck

Power

Protection

Chakras

The third chakra (Solar plexus)

The Sacral Chakra

The Throat Chakra

Amethyst

Amethyst is a semi-precious type of Quartz crystal found in a number of places around the world and primarily occurs in hues from a light pink/violet to deep purple and blue, sometimes even appearing to have secondary red hues. The name Amethyst comes from the geek word ametusthos which means 'not intoxicated' and throughout history, it has enjoyed the special virtue of preventing drunkenness and overindulgence. It has been said that an Amethyst worn at navel level will bring about soberness and control over indulgent thoughts, whilst keeping Amethyst anywhere on your person could increase intelligence and even inspire shrewd business decisions.

Purple Amethyst, in particular, has always been held in high esteem throughout the ages due to its remarkable beauty and ability to boost, soothe, and stimulate our emotions and the energy fields surrounding our bodies. In earlier history, Amethyst was regarded as one of the most valuable of the Precious Stones, however, in recent times due to large deposits being located in areas such as Brazil, Serbia and Sri Lanka. Sometimes known as the 'stone of spirit', Amethyst is typically the same colour as the crown chakra (our doorway to the divine) and is traditionally used in the making of Mala beads in Tibet which are an ancient meditation tool said to aid in the realignment of the chakra network as well as having calming and cleansing effects on the spirit. Amethyst is also known as the Bishop's Stone and is still worn by Bishops today, sometimes in the form of the episcopal ring, in this case, the Amethyst represents piety, humility, wisdom, and an allusion to the old adage of the Apostles as 'not drunk'. The protective powers of Amethyst have been alluded to throughout the ages; the stone has been used as protection against all manner of witchcraft and even night terrors and nightmares, with the Egyptians using the gemstone to ward against feelings of fear and guilt. Amethyst is regarded as one of the 'Power Stones' and has long been associated with wisdom, the preservation of wisdom and of psychic and spiritual healing. Often referred to as the best gemstone for anxiety, Amethyst soothes and relaxes the nervous system and is commonly used to combat the negative effects of stress and even cure headaches. Amethyst is a go-to gemstone regularly worn by healers of all types due to its ability to focus positive and healing energies and works especially well when set within silver jewellery.

Colour

Purple/Lilac/Violet, with possible light pinkish or deeper blue hues

Birthstone

February

Zodiac

Aries

Aquarius

Capricorn

Pisces

Planet

Saturn

Energetic Frequencies

Healing

Power

Protection

Chakras

The seventh or Crown Chakra (Pineal gland)

Apatite

Apatite received its name as a derivative of the Greek word meaning 'to deceive', mainly due to the array of different colours in which Apatite chooses to manifest. It is a multi-faceted gemstone that is usually blue but also brown, yellow, and green. Apatite holds several favourable properties such as aiding the body in absorbing calcium which in turn strengthens bones, cartilage, teeth, soothes joints and helps with issues connected to hypertension. This is a stone that boosts motor skills and creativity in all its forms, however, some colours, in particular, carry their own meanings and energetic frequencies separate from 'common' Apatite.

Blue Apatite

Blue Apatite is well known as an inspirational stone, helping those who wear it to fine tune their natural communication skills and powers of self-expression and often used by those hoping to practice and develop their latent psychic abilities. This spiritual gemstone is renowned for cleansing the aura and it is said that Blue Apatite has a particular synchronicity with the energetic frequencies contained within the legendary Akashic records. Blue Apatite is intrinsically linked to the Throat Chakra and tuned into the energies of the Third Eye which boosts both concentration and memory making it a highly valuable talisman for communicators of all kinds from business consultants and marketers to public speakers and teachers. Blue Apatite allows for direct psychic contact with our astral/true/finer/inner self where we will perceive hidden knowledge and release all negative energy.

Yellow or Golden Apatite

Yellow or Golden Apatite is a Fire Element Stone which has the dual uses of boosting both intellect and power in order to achieve personal goals. Clear Yellow Apatite is one of the purest gemstones, emanating energy, not unlike that of a sunny disposition that acts to provide us with feelings of clarity, self-esteem and self-worth. This 'Solar Stone' is associated with masculine energy and can aid the indecisive in becoming more assertive or even providing the wearer with the courage to combat anxious feelings in order to help them through challenging situations. It is also known as a 'Learning Stone' increasing the focus and concentration of the user whilst simultaneously purging any listlessness, leaving the user invigorated, motivated and ready to hit the books. Yellow Apatite is associated with the Solar Plexus Chakra and is great for dislodging any negative energy blockages within the body's Chakra Network alleviating the user from feeling of lethargy or depression and is also known to stimulate our action centres which are located at the centre of the Navel Chakra which in turns provides us with overwhelming feelings of hope.

Green Apatite

Known in Spain as 'The Asparagus stone' Green Apatite is well known for its ability to balance the wisdom of the mind with the intuition and love of the heart in order to allow the wearer to ascertain the best possible course of action. It is a gemstone commonly used by healers the world over to assist them by providing a clean and clear energy which is conducive to the healing process. Being closely associated with both wisdom and nature Green Apatite is thought to facilitate the user in communicating with the nature spirit or even delving into past life regressions. Green Apatite is a fitting talisman for those feeling tired or suffering from 'burnout' as the lively energy that radiates from Green Apatite can re-ignite long lost enthusiasm and refocus our efforts in personal projects and long-term goals. Green Apatite aids in cell growth and regeneration and is renowned for helping dieters maintain stable eating patterns and a healthy diet by removing negative feelings anxiety and stress, this allows us to realign our actions with the intentions of our higher self.

Colour

Blue

Yellow

Green/Brown

Birthstone

December

Planet

Ketu

Energetic Frequencies

Motivation

Power

Healing

Chakras

The Throat Chakra (blue)

The Solar Plexus Chakra (golden/yellow)

The Navel Chakra (golden/yellow)

Heart Chakra (green)

Chapter 3: Understanding The Chakras And Their Connection To Crystal Healing

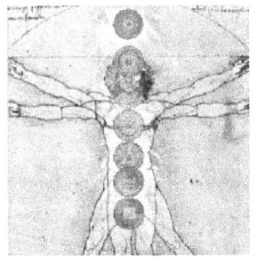

Crystals can heal anything from a broken heart to intense migraines. Also, using crystals while practicing meditation enhances the power of meditation. Crystals help in aligning the seven primary chakras in your body and ensure that the energy levels are balanced in each chakra. Let us look at the seven chakras, their purpose in the body, and how crystals can help in stabilizing them.

So, what are chakras? They are energy centers within and close to the human body that regulate all biological, chemical, and emotional processes taking place inside us. These energy centers or chakras are responsible for proper functioning of all aspects of the human body ranging from the simplest and smallest organ to the most complex immune system.

There are seven primary chakras positioned all over our body starting from the base of the spine right up to the crown of the human head. Each chakra has its own unique vibrational energy, color, and energy frequency associated with it. At this juncture, it makes sense to reiterate the fact that the human body is also a form of energy. The efficient functioning of your energy centers is vital for your body and mind to function optimally which, in turn, keeps you emotionally, psychologically, spiritually, and physically balanced.

In Sanskrit, chakra translates to 'wheel.' These colored wheels are represented as continuously spinning so as to maintain energy balance in your body. The concept of chakras is believed to have originated in India more than 3500 years ago, around 1500 B.C. However, this novel idea was taken to the West only in the 20th century.

The Seven Chakras and Their Significance

Let us look at the seven chakras, their locations in the human body, and their functions.

The root chakra (Mooladhara) - This chakra is located at the base of the spine, and the color associated with it is red. The root chakra is responsible for survival and grounding issues. Survival issues include food, clothing, shelter, money, wealth, financial independence, etc. When these basic survival needs are met, then you feel secure and grounded.

The root chakra is the starting point of our development. The spine begins its development from the bottom and moves up toward the crown. The root chakra is associated with basic survival questions such as 'Do I belong on this earth and to the family into which I was born?' The mooladhara represents the primal, animal nature of human beings.

The root chakra governs the primal survival energy like the fight, flight, and freeze responses. This chakra forms the basis of our life force energy and connects our energy system with that of the physical world. The organs that are governed by the root chakra include the kidneys, adrenal glands, colon, bones, arterial blood flow from the left side of the heart to the rest of the body, and muscles.

A root chakra that functions well gives the motivation necessary to sleep, eat, and live well. It helps in the development of self-esteem, personal integrity, and provides us with a sense of belonging. As the name suggests, the root chakra helps us connect to the earth by rooting ourselves.

A blocked root chakra results in loss of vitality even our zest for life can be significantly compromised. An unbalanced root chakra can take away your sense of belonging resulting in a feeling of being lost and lonely. Consequently, we feel restless, anxious, depressed, resentful and frustrated.

The energy of the root chakra facilitates the development of courage and resourcefulness empowering us to live well and to the best of our abilities even during challenging times. This chakra is also the densest of all the seven, which is the reason why the color red is attributed to it.

Red is the most stimulating color and also the one with the longest and slowest wavelength. Red is also the color of blood, the first color that we come in contact with when we are born. The color of the root chakra demands attention and signals danger to us.

The sacral chakra (Svadhisthana) - This chakra is the center of your pleasure, passion, sexuality, and creativity. It is associated with intimacy, feelings, sensuality, and connections with people. Located in the pelvic area, the sacral chakra is not satisfied with mere survival like the root chakra. The Svadhisthana seeks pleasure and enjoyment.

The power of this chakra lies in its ability to help us experience life fully through our senses and emotions. The energy vibration of the sacral chakra allows you to let go and accept the changes and transformations in your life as they happen. It allows you to experience and engage with life fully and uninhibitedly.

One of the biggest challenges of balancing the sacral chakra lies in the way our society has developed. In most of the 'culturally accepted' and 'civilized' societies, emotions are almost always relegated to the background. Manifesting emotions is considered uncivilized and expressing emotions is frowned upon as being shameful and uncultured.

We are trained to 'control' our emotions and feelings. Repeated and consistent disconnections with our emotions make us lose touch with ourselves, and we find ways and means to suppress our feelings even further. This approach results in the unbalancing of the sacral chakra.

Also, the Svadhisthana is the center of creativity, and passion fuels creativity. All your creations ranging from a simple poem to conceiving a child and everything in between originate in the sacral chakra. An individual with a clear sacral chakra is passionate and does not hesitate to live his or her life meaningfully and with fulfillment. Signs of a blocked or unbalanced sacral chakra include:

- Lack of motivation and creativity
- Persistent breakdown of relationships
- Low libido

- Emotional confusion and upheavals
- Lack of self-esteem and a feeling of being unloved
- Lack of self-care

Orange is the color of the Svadhisthana, and orange-hued crystals are great for balancing and clearing energy blocks of this chakra.

The solar plexus chakra (Manipura) - This chakra facilitates the ability to radiate your power to the world. It represents your mental faculties, personal power, and expression of will. A well-functioning solar plexus chakra allows us to assert ourselves to the outside world. The Sanskrit word 'Manipura' translates to 'city of jewels' or 'city of gems.'

Located in the upper part of the stomach, the solar plexus chakra is the third one counting from the bottom, and is very closely connected with our digestive system. One of the main functions of the solar plexus is to convert matter into energy for effective use by the human body and mind. This chakra also governs the functioning of the pancreas and manages and regulates metabolism.

Other vital responsibilities and areas of governance of this chakra include:

- Will and personal power
- Self-responsibility
- Intellectual and mental capabilities
- Decision-making and clarity of judgments
- Personality and personal identity
- Self-discipline, self-confidence
- Independence

This energy center provides the momentum you need to take your dreams forward and realize them. It guides your life purpose and acts like a compass ensuring you are moving ahead to your destined destination. It also influences your self-image and social status.

When the solar plexus clear is clear and open, the emotions related to these human functions find a good outlet empowering you to manifest your capabilities in the best way possible, and consequently achieve self-actualization. Any state of imbalance or energy blockages in Manipura can result in negative symptoms in your emotional, spiritual, and mental realms. Here are some signs that reflect an unbalanced or blocked solar plexus chakra:

- Excessive authority or control over the people and things around you

- Feeling of helplessness, rashness, and irresponsibility

- A deep desire for manipulation and misuse of power

- Lack of purpose and direction

- Lack of decision-making and planning capabilities

Yellow is the color associated with this chakra, and rightly so, because the nature element associated with the solar plexus chakra is fire. In some cases, this chakra is represented in a yellowish-red color too.

The heart chakra (Anahata) - The heart chakra has the power to fill our lives with beauty, love, compassion and joy. The working of this chakra is driven by the principles of integration and transformation. It serves as a bridge between our materialistic and spiritual aspirations.

Located right in the middle of the chest between the breasts, the heart chakra is the fourth one after the solar plexus chakra, and is related to the element of air. Interestingly, the heart chakra is situated slightly to the left of our physical heart. It is associated with breathing and the movement of air within our body. The organs governed by the heart chakra include the lungs and the cardiac system as these organs are dependent on each other as well as on air for proper functioning. The heart chakra is also related to spaciousness and connectivity between things and people. The energy of this chakra is multidimensional.

This chakra also governs the functioning of the thymus gland and regulation of the immune system. The primary aspects controlled and managed by the heart chakra are:

• Self-love and love for others

• Relationships - experiencing meaningful and deep relationships

• Transcending the limitations of ego

• Appreciating the beauty of all things around us

• Forgiveness, compassion, acceptance, and empathy

• Changes and transformations

- Ability to achieve peace and calmness by overcoming grief

- Self-awareness and insight

Additionally, the heart chakra connects the lower and upper chakras, which is the reason this energy center is responsible for the integration of earthly and spiritual matter of our lives. The heart chakra is capable of perceiving the energies of all the chakras blending harmoniously. Therefore, Anahata is all about connecting and relating with an emphasis on giving and taking with an open heart and mind.

Also, love is a powerful emotion with the power to positively transform emotions and life experiences. There can be no real relationship in the absence of love. It is crucial to remember that love in this context is not limited to just the romantic feeling between lovers but includes all kinds of love between human beings. Love also helps to overcome limitations of ego.

When the heart chakra is opened, balanced, and unblocked, we are able to live a life of love and compassion helping us become self-aware in any situation. When the heart chakra is not functioning at its most efficient levels, then you are likely to experience one or more of the following symptoms:

- You feel defensive about everything in your life

- You feel a sense of being closed and trapped

- You are scared of intimacy and also feel jealous about others and their achievements

- You feel excessively codependent which means you need the approval of others to feel and be happy

- You feel compelled to be a savior or rescuer or a victim in all situations in your life. You lack objectivity

- You become antisocial and reclusive

- You hold grudges, and you find it difficult to forgive and let go

Green is the color associated with the heart chakra although in certain high-frequency energies, it can turn pink, which is the reason why the heart chakra and love are associated with the color pink.

The throat chakra (Vishuddha) - The fifth chakra is located at the center of the neck in line with the throat. This chakra allows for the smooth flow of energy between the head and the lower parts of the body. The function of the throat chakra is connected to communication and expression.

The Sanskrit term for the throat chakra is Vishuddha, which translates to 'pure.' This chakra is related to the element of sound. The principle of sound that governs the throat chakra is the idea that the sound emanating from the throat gets propagated through the air. The influence of this sound vibration is not just felt by the ears but by the entire body.

The body parts governed by the throat chakra include jaws, mouth, pharynx, tongue, palate, neck and shoulders. The gland connected to this chakra is the thyroid gland. The energy of the throat chakra regulates the body energy by controlling metabolism, body temperature, and cellular growth. Some of the primary functions of the throat chakra are:

- Expression, especially to your ability of speaking the truth

- All kinds of communication including verbal, nonverbal, external, and internal

- Connecting and communicating with subtle realms like the spiritual space and intuition

- Ability to articulate thoughts and ideas clearly and convincingly

- Finding your purpose and vocation

- Providing a strong sense of time

The throat chakra is all about expressing yourself and your purpose to the world. Interestingly, the throat chakra has a natural connection with the sacral chakra that deals with creativity and emotion. After all, the throat chakra's primary job is to empower you to articulate your creativity in its most authentic form.

Sitting just below the chakras of the head, the throat chakra can also help you connect yourself with the spiritual realm. Opening the throat chakra and unblocking it can help in releasing pressures and stresses accumulated in the lower heart chakra. The signs of an unbalanced throat chakra are:

- Speaking excessively or inadequately; basically, no control over your speech.
- Lack of listening skills
- Fear of speaking

- Small and very soft voice that can hardly be heard
- Inability to keep secrets and promises
- Telling lies
- Excessively shy or secretive
- No sense of direction and purpose

The color associated with the throat chakra is turquoise blue or aquamarine blue. Sometimes, the color purple is also used to represent this chakra.

The third eye chakra (Ajna chakra) - Located between the brows on the forehead, the third eye chakra is the epicenter of intuition and foresight. This chakra works on the power of imagination and openness.

The Sanskrit word for the third eye chakra is 'Ajna' which translates to 'command' and 'seeing.' According to ancient Hindu beliefs, the power of the third eye rests in its ability to help you transcend your dual nature and connect you with the supreme universal power.

The pineal gland, which regulates and controls the biorhythms (including the circadian rhythm) of the body is governed by the third eye chakra. This gland, which is located in the brain, is also connected with the effect of light (as it is situated close to the optic nerve) and perception. This gland is believed to regulate the mystical states of consciousness. The main functions of the third eye chakra include:

- Vision and intuition

- Perceiving subtle energy movements and dimensions

- Psychic abilities like clairvoyance

- Access to mystical states of consciousness

- Related to insight and wisdom

- Develops inspiration and creativity

The Ajna Chakra goes beyond the physical realm of human existence and allows you to connect with the energy realms. When your third eye is open, your intuitive powers and inner perceptions are enhanced. The third eye chakra helps us see things differently and, therefore, describing your perceptions in physical terms or through the usual channels of human communication can be difficult. You have to necessarily experience it to understand it.

Most of the visions seen through the third eye chakra are 'ghost-like' or 'blurry.' However, if you are deeply connected to this energy center, then you can see things like in a movie. Building this capability requires you to practice relaxation methods that are different from the usual way of resting that you are used to. It requires repeated and persistent practice before an average person can access the limitless powers of this chakra. An imbalanced third eye chakra can manifest in one or more of the following ways:

• You feel stuck in the daily grind and are not able to perceive things beyond your mundane existence

• An overactive third eye might make you live in a fantasy world instead of accepting the real world

• You find it difficult to visualize your future and are unable to find ways and means to reach your potential

• You tend to reject everything connected to spirituality and superhuman capabilities

• You find it difficult to see the bigger picture in any given situation

• Lack of clarity

The color of this chakra is purple or bluish purple although certain energy frequencies can be seen as bluish white or translucent purple. This chakra is more connected to the soft radiance it emits which reminds us of moonlight than the color.

The crown chakra (Sahasrara) - Located at the top of your head, the crown chakra is the seventh and the last of the primary chakras within the human body. This chakra gives us access to the higher states of consciousness, and is powered by the universal consciousness.

The Sanskrit word for the crown chakra is Sahasrara, which translates to 'a thousand petals.' This chakra sits like a crown on or slightly above your head radiating its energy outward. The pituitary gland is governed by the crown chakra although it oversees the functions of the pineal and hypothalamus glands too. Considering that this chakra is located on our heads, it is closely related to the functioning of the brain and nervous system.

The energies of the first (root) chakra and the last (crown) chakra are connected as they lie in the extremities of the chakra line. The primary psychological and physical functions controlled and governed by the crown chakra are:

- Wisdom and consciousness

- Everything that is considered sacred

- Connection with the limitless and formless universal energy

- Realization and freedom from the limitations of physical things

- Connection with the higher states of consciousness

- Ecstasy and bliss

The crown chakra is connected with breaking and transcending all limitations associated with time and space. When you open the crown chakra, you get access to the limitless aspect of the universe. If and when you connect with your crown chakra, you feel a blissful union with the entire universe resulting in spiritual ecstasy. The crown chakra helps you access the power of enlightened wisdom and utmost clarity of thought. An imbalanced or blocked crown chakra can be manifested in the following ways:

- You feel disconnected with spirituality

- You are constantly in a cynical mood

- An overactive crown chakra can make you feel disconnected from your body

- You could feel obsessively connected to all spiritual matters

- You could feel close-minded

The color of the Sahasrara is white although sometimes, it is represented by a deep shade of purple too.

Balancing and Healing the Chakras with Crystals

Each time a chakra becomes unbalanced, overactive, or underactive, the functionality of those aspects connected to that particular chakra goes awry throwing your life out of control. Therefore, it is imperative that you make sure all your chakra energies are balanced. There are multiple ways of balancing and cleansing your chakras. Some of the most popular methods include:

- Mindful breathing and other mindfulness exercises
- Reiki
- Tai chi
- Yoga
- Acupuncture and acupressure
- Aromatherapy

Another extremely popular method used to balance chakras is through crystal healing. Each chakra is associated with a particular color and specific crystals. These cleansed and cleaned stones are placed on the relevant body part so that the matching vibrational frequency of the crystals correct misaligned energy frequencies in the chakra. Consequently, the energy in the chakras gets balanced and associated functionalities are restored to normalcy. Let us look at the chakras again along with their corresponding crystals.

The root chakra - Healing the root chakra with crystals clears the negative energies and also gets rid of energy blockages. The color of the root chakra is red and the crystals that heal this energy center include:

Red carnelian - Red carnelian crystals are effective healers of the root chakra. Wearing a bracelet or ring with a red carnelian will help in clearing out negative energies in the root chakra right through the day.

Tourmaline - Black tourmaline is excellent for healing the root chakra. In addition to healing the base chakra, black tourmaline balances the meridian connecting the root chakra to the crown chakra and passing through all the ones in between.

Garnet - Red garnet, almandine, pyrope, and andradite are excellent healing crystals for the root chakra. Red garnet especially keeps your energetic right through the day even as it continually clears impurities. Seven drops of red garnet elixir twice a day is an excellent remedy for root chakra imbalances and energy blockages.

The sacral chakra - The color of the sacral chakra is orange and the crystals that work very well for this energy center include:

Orange carnelian - The energy alignment of orange carnelian is in perfect sync with that of the sacral chakra, and it is, therefore, an excellent crystal for healing this energy center. Using this crystal for healing helps you improve your instincts and 'gut feel' while bolstering your intuitive powers.

Yellow and golden citrine - Healing with yellow and golden citrine improves your decision-making capabilities even as your creativity and energy levels get a big boost.

Spessartine garnet - This is a special kind of garnet that promises to bring alive your creative, sexual, and artistic talents. In fact, the power of spessartine garnet is so strong that excessive use of this crystal could be a bit overwhelming. So, it makes sense to restrict wearing only a couple of small crystals in your bracelet or a little tumble stone.

Tiger's eye - In addition to revving up your sexual energy, the tiger's eye crystal delivers emotional, spiritual, and physical balance.

When you start using crystals to heal your sacral chakra, it is likely that you will see blotches of orange color wherever you go for some time. There is nothing to be alarmed about in this. It is a common occurrence that is experienced by most people during the initial stages of sacral chakra healing.

The solar plexus chakra - Yellow-colored crystals vibrate in consonance with the frequency of the solar plexus energy center and, therefore, are great for healing that energy center. Here are some excellent healing crystals for the solar plexus chakra:

Citrine - This yellow or golden crystal clears your third chakra and allows it to be healed very quickly and effectively.

Tiger's eye - This crystal is a powerful healer of the solar plexus chakra. Cleansing and clearing your third chakra with the tiger's eye crystal makes you feel balanced and powerful.

Golden-yellow labradorite - Also known as sunstone and bytownite, the golden-yellow labradorite helps clear the energy blockages in the solar plexus chakra and helps in building confidence, vitality, and assertiveness.

Peridot - This beautiful olive green gemstone is great for cleansing and activating the powers of the solar plexus as well as the heart chakra. It is a little tricky to work with and requires some amount of practice and skill.

The heart chakra - Numerous crystals for healing and cleansing the heart chakra are available for you. Resonating at the right frequency to match the energy of the heart chakra, these crystals absorb negative ions and tune up the chakra for optimal efficiency and functioning. When you use these heart chakra healing crystals, you are bound to notice and experience the following positive symptoms:

• The tightness in your chest created by blocked energy as well as the accumulation of negative energy will clear. Your chest will expand, and suddenly you will feel that you are able to breathe far more freely than before.

• Your relationships with people in your personal and professional life will see a significant improvement.

- You will enjoy interacting with other people and find that your level of patience has gone up.

You can use any of the following green or pink crystals to heal and cleanse your heart chakra:

Green aventurine - This green crystal has the power to soothe and calm your heart chakra and empower you with harmony and balance. Green aventurine is known for its power to improve your romantic relationships.

Rose quartz - This beautiful rose-colored crystal improves the clarity of your thought and empowers you with making better judgmental calls, especially in the realm of personal relationships.

Aquamarine - This beautiful crystal soothes, cleanses, and activates the energy vibrations of the heart and throat chakras. A challenging aspect of this crystal is that it could reveal certain hidden personal truths about yourself and your life that you may not be ready to accept. Therefore, in the initial stages, it is wise to restrict the use of aquamarine to not more than 5-10 minutes.

Olive-green and pale-green peridot - Helping in promoting balance and harmony throughout your body, these two green crystals are excellent for healing your heart chakra. Peridot is specifically prescribed for those times when you are trying to recover from the loss of a relationship or a loved one.

The throat chakra - Here are some crystals that work best for the healing of the throat chakra:

Lapis lazuli - This beautiful blue crystal is great for stimulation, opening, and balancing of the throat chakra energies. It restores your lost or forgotten communication skills and capabilities.

Amazonite - This green/turquoise-green crystal destroys and protects the user from negative powers even as it restores balance and harmony.

Aquamarine - This blue-green crystal is great for stimulation of positive energy in the throat chakra. It provides courage and strength while helping you get rid of fear and uncertainty even as you develop tolerance and compassion.

Turquoise - Perfect for balance and stimulation, turquoise is a crystal that works very well to heal the throat chakra. It builds your confidence to speak out the truth and articulate your thoughts confidently and without fear.

The third eye chakra - You could use any of the following crystals and gemstones for healing and cleansing your third eye chakra:

Moldavite - This dark green crystal is used to stimulate, balance, and cleanse your third eye chakra. In addition to clearing the negativity from your sixth chakra, Moldavite works to restore balance in the entire chakra system. This crystal is great for dream recall, to see new perspectives, and to increase dreams.

Amethyst - This stone, which is available in varying shades of purple, provides powers to gain wisdom, protection from harm, and healing powers too.

Black obsidian - This crystal is great for dispelling negative energies as well as to balance the energy of the third eye chakra. It also helps improve emotional control.

Purple fluorite - This purple gemstone promotes mental clarity, intuition, and your powers of concentration.

The crown chakra - The following stones are great for cleansing, balancing and clearing energy blockages in the crown chakra:

Selenite - Selenite is a clear, crystalline gemstone that opens and stimulates the crown chakra. Clearing congested energies, it also dispels negativity in the auric field. Meditating while wearing or holding a jewel with selenite can lift you to higher states of consciousness.

Clear quartz - This wondrous crystal is empowered with reprogrammable memory. It also amplifies the energy of your crown chakra. It is helpful to expand consciousness, bring in heightened spiritual awareness, and opens up the crown chakra. It facilitates connecting with spiritual guides.

Diamond - This highly precious gemstone has access to divine energies, and if used persistently, can take you to higher levels of consciousness. It promotes your honesty and truth and also clears emotional blockages in your body and mind.

Chakras and crystals are closely related and are interdependent for optimal use of their auric fields and powers. While there are other ways to clear and cleanse the energy fields of your chakras, using crystals is doubly effective because you can access the powerful energy of the crystals as well.

Chapter 4: Which Crystals Should I Use?

Now the next question: How do you select your gemstones? There are so many crystals out there of various cuts, colors, and shapes. Each characteristic has a corresponding purpose. In the end, your choice of stones will depend greatly on whether you have a specific issue that you wish to resolve.

Crystal Shapes

Arrowheads

This shape is often noted in black obsidian. Arrowheads are perfect particularly for people who require a constant reminder that there is always a direction that can guide their decisions and their destinations.

Geodes

These pertain to round rock formations commonly seen in amethyst, agate, and quartz. When broken open, geodes reveal a lovely crystalline interior. This particular shape is great for those who desire to be more grounded during moments of contemplation.

Hearts

Heart shaped gemstones are often used to address areas that are governed by the heart chakra. Use heart-shaped crystals when resolving issues pertaining to love and relationships or when you want to invite romance into your life.

Pyramids

These crystals may come in triangle, pentagon, or square varieties. They are considered as polyhedrons, that is, they all have three dimensions, level bases, and straight edges. This type of shape is recommended for those who wish to increase their concentration and preservation of knowledge and wisdom. Pyramids also bring about protection.

Spheres

Spherical shaped crystals appear as balls or orbs and this is the most preferable shape when you wish to attain unity with life. Spheres are also great to use during meditation.

Cubes

Cubical crystals are often utilized for matters involving the completion of a life cycle. You may also use cube-shaped crystals in situations where you are hoping for the best results.

Octahedrons

These are three-dimensional shapes which consist of 8 symmetrical triangular planes. Octahedrons are often used to achieve steadiness and internal strength. Whenever you come across a huge responsibility at work or in the domestic setting, use this stone shape.

Clusters

These are made up of small crystals that have naturally fused together. They are often used for the purposes of cleansing, invigorating, and calming the environment. Its design symbolizes the interconnectedness of all beings. As such, cluster-shaped crystals tend to be useful when your intentions have broad umbrella effects.

Wands

This type of shape can be achieved naturally although some manufacturers tend to fashion some stones in this form as well. Wand-shaped crystals are ideal for people who wish to enhance their memory and intensify their concentration. Wand-shaped stones also help to add vitality.

Various Healing Crystals and their Purposes

The **Amazonite** is perfect for individuals who are currently going through a tough emotional process. This gemstone has a soothing effect and aids in allaying anxiety and fear. It is recommended for individuals with neurological problems.

The **Amber** also yields a calming effect. Likewise, it helps to refresh your energy.

The **Amethyst** is effective in dispelling negative thoughts and in retraining your brain to think positively. It also helps relieve emotional blockages. It enhances your sensibility and assists you in moving towards a more conscious state. Furthermore, it is useful for people suffering from migraine and arthritis. Placing an amethyst on your desk will allow you to think at your highest level.

The **Apache Tear** is advised if you are currently suffering from loss and grief. It is useful in breaking down emotional barriers and thus, is helpful in cases where you need to forgive and let go.

The **Aquamarine** works to cure phobias and helps a person to achieve stability.

Use the **Aventurine** if you want to purify your body and your emotions. As previously mentioned, this gemstone is often used in healing baths to help you achieve tranquility.

The **Bloodstone** is good for grounding and for providing support during emotional situations.

The **Blue Lace Agate** is handy in relieving emotional and spiritual tension.

Meanwhile, the **Botswana Agate** is suggested for people who are in the habit of smoking. This will also aid you in managing and expressing repressed emotions.

All colors of **Calcite** are great cleansers for your chakras. Use these stones if you wish to be able to move on after a devastating emotional upset. The blue calcite is particularly used for calming a racing heartbeat.

The **Carnelian** may be used as a protection against envy. It enables you to connect with your higher self and thus prevents you from being victims of negative emotions like sorrow, anger, and fear. This stone is helpful in chasing away apathy and it also aids in fostering trust. This is accomplished by linking your inferior chakras (sacral, solar plexus, etc.) to your heart chakra.

For those who are seeking emotional release, the **Celestite** may be used.

Meanwhile, choose to invest in a **Chrysocolla** is you're after emotional strength. This gemstone also helps in providing you with relief from guilt.

The **Chrysoprase** healing stone is for individuals suffering from alcoholism and depression. The stone can help provide you with energy and patience to work on the small changes and to take the recovery process one baby step at a time.

If it is happiness that you wish for, then the **Citrine** is what you should invest in. It encourages spontaneous expression and helps you get rid of your fears. It is often called the "Success Stone" because it provides the bearer with a more positive outlook and attracts prosperity. If you wish to invite more money, place a citrine crystal inside your wallet.

The **Clear Quartz** is great for converting negative energy to positive energy. It is best used as a pendant because it can help deflect harmful radiation away from your body. Writers who are suffering from "the block" can boost their creativity by staring at clear quartz for a few minutes.

Emerald gemstones allow you to keep in line with your purpose in life.

All shades of the **Fluorite** can be used to calm your emotions.

The **Hematite** is most popularly known as the "Anti-stress Stone". When someone throws negative energy at you, this crystal sends all that negative energy back to the sender. To enhance electromagnetic circulation, attach a small piece of this stone onto your back.

The **Hemimorphite** is useful in shielding your vulnerable self-esteem and it also helps your intentions to grow more pure. Use this stone if you have a tendency to harbor negative feelings and anger towards others.

The **Kunzite** provides the carrier with a sense of well-being as well as a sense of mental peace.

Lapis lazuli is effective in providing mental clarity and in maintaining objectivity. It also promotes self-acceptance.

The **Larimar** helps eliminate feelings of impending doom, which are frequently experienced by people who are suffering from anxiety attacks.

Meanwhile, the **Lepidolite** minimizes stress responses and eliminates feelings of hopelessness. This gemstone is also used to treat insomnia.

The **Malachite** is often used together with the rose quartz in healing broken hearts. It is perfect for type A personalities and for individuals who are at risk for suffering from internal organ diseases.

The **Moonstone** is suggested for people who lack emotional nurturing.

The **Moss Agate** is best for soothing wounded self-esteems and egos that have been badly hurt. It also cultivates your strengths.

The **Obsidian** is an extremely powerful crystal that has the capacity to overpower old energy patterns. Energy blockages are converted into white light.

The **Onyx** has the power to absorb your grief and to relieve you from your mental confusion.

The **Opal**, on the other hand, is great for driving out dark moods. Use it for periods of discernment and during quests for the truth.

If you're suffering from jealousy, you might benefit from the powers of the **Peridot**. It helps in overcoming self-centered ideas as well as self-destructive thoughts.

The **Petrified Wood** is another type of crystal which comes highly recommended for people who are naturally nervous and those who have a tendency to worry a lot.

The **Rhodocrosite** allows you to balance your emotions after encountering moments of severe stress.

The **Rose Quartz** is popularly used in providing loving comfort to the bearer. It is often called the "Love Stone". To allow yourself to relax after a stressful day, place the rose quartz on your heart chakra for 15 minutes.

Those who are seeking to move past their emotional states to transcend towards higher psycho-spiritual centers will benefit from the **Selenite** crystal.

The **Smoky Quartz** is perfect for those who stubbornly refuse to let go of negativity in their life. It can stabilize your mood swings and absorb and convert negative energy. If you know someone who's cranky, stressed out, burned out, or is suffering from PMS, this gemstone can be an ideal gift.

The **Snakeskin Agate** promotes cheerfulness.

The **Sodalite** helps in subduing mental noise,

The **Tiger Eye** is for people who are having trouble with handling responsibility.

Meanwhile, the **Pink Tourmaline** is effective for people who are seeking protection from victimization. It also provides the wearer with a sense of great beauty.

The **Turquoise** enables the bearer to achieve a degree of emotional detachment, thus enabling him to concentrate on self-accomplishment without being distracted by others. It is popularly known as the "Protection Stone". When worn on the throat chakra, it helps improve one's communication skills and guides him in speaking the truth. Furthermore, this gemstone is used to prevent premature aging.

The **Unakite** come in two colors. The Pink Unakite is connected with movement and the Green Unakite is connected with grounding. This gemstone helps the person move on after suffering from a severe disappointment.

Chapter 5: Crystals For Everyone

Crystals aren't racist, sexist, religious zealots or biased in any way. Things like age and personality don't matter, and anyone willing to put in the time and effort can try crystal healing. The only prerequisites are an open mind and a very basic understanding of how to apply crystal healing, since simply buying a healing crystal isn't going to change your life. Crystals are fairly easy to come by, and always ready to improve your life. Unfortunately, crystals can be picky at times. Different types of crystal resonate better with different people. A crystal that works miracles for me, may not work for you at all. This is because the energy in a crystal simply doesn't react well to the energy inside your body. This can be a big factor in why many people dismiss crystal healing as a fantasy: they try a very basic recipe for "how to fix a certain problem with this specific crystal" and end up gaining no effects simply because the crystal doesn't resonate with them. There are many crystals with similar effects and abilities, so if one crystal does not work for you, try different crystals with similar properties until you find something that works for you. Choosing a crystal that resonates well with your own energy is especially important when the crystal is meant to be worn for long periods of time, but more on choosing crystals a little later.

Birthstones

This is a system that allocates specific crystals and gemstones to the months of the year. It is a fairly old concept that has undergone some changes, but the current tradition is to give someone a birthstone corresponding with the month they are born in. Birthstones are usually worn as a piece of jewelry, and for many people, birthstones are their first introduction to crystals. Many believe this system found its origins with Aaron's breastplate, which is mentioned in the book of Exodus in the bible. This breastplate was studded with twelve gemstones to represent the twelve tribes of Israel, and different interpretations of old texts determined which gemstones these would be, and each was assigned a month of the year. In the eighth and ninth century B.C. the Christian church assigned a stone to each of the twelve apostles, and the custom was to own a set of twelve birthstones and wear each stone during the month assigned to them. This was done in an attempt to honor the apostles and as a teaching method for children to help remember their names. The custom of wearing only the stone assigned to your own month is a much more modern concept that can be dated back to somewhere between the 1500s to the 1800s. These birthstones varied due to different translations and interpretations, but a general pattern could be detected. In 1912, the American National Association of Jewelers put together a standard list of birthstones, which has now become the global standard. There is very little correspondence to historical origins or crystal abilities and symbolism in this list, and many believe this specific list to be little more than a sales pitch. There have been many different cultures around the world that used the birthstone concept, each with their own personal touches. The Chinese culture, as an example, assigns the stones to the twelve zodiac signs rather than the months.

Another system of birthstones uses a color wheel that indicates colors associated with the different time of the year, and associates crystals of the same color to the twelve months. This color wheel system uses a much more accurate approach in terms of symbology, psychology and a study of the use of talismans throughout history to determine which crystal types are more suited to a person based on the time of year they were born in. This system can be a good place to start when you're looking to buy your first healing crystal and want to find something that resonates well with you. Here is a list of the crystal color types that are associated with the different months and some examples:

- 21 Dec to 19 Jan - violet-colored crystals like amethyst, purple agate, and fluorite

- 20 Jan to 18 Feb - indigo-colored crystals like tanzanite, sodalite, and lapis lazuli

- 19 Feb to 19 Mar - blue-colored crystals like aquamarine, blue agate, and kyanite

- 20 Mar to 19 Apr - turquoise-colored crystals like turquoise, and some variants of aquamarine and agate

- 20 Apr to 20 May - green-colored crystals like emerald, alexandrite, and jade

- 21 May to 20 Jun - olive-colored crystals like prehnite and pyromorphite

- 21 Jun to 21 Jul - yellow-colored crystals like citrine, yellow apatite, and cat's eye

- 22 Jul to 21 Aug - gold-colored crystals like golden beryl and cat's eye

- 22 Aug to 22 Sep - orange-colored crystals like amber, carnelian, and sunstone

- 23 Sep to 21 Oct - scarlet-colored crystals like red emerald and red beryl

- 22 Oct to 20 Nov - red-colored crystals like ruby, red jasper, and garnet

- 21 Nov to 20 Dec - amethyst-colored crystals like cacoxenite

Crystal Healing for Children

Any parent will tell you that the question they ask the most is "Is this safe for my child?" In this case, the answer is yes. Crystal healing is perfectly safe for children and should be encouraged, as they are perfect for crystal healing. Children experience the same effects as adults when working with crystals and are naturally more open and susceptible to the energy emitted by crystals, meaning the effects are stronger on them than adults. They are almost always fascinated by crystals and are willing to simply believe in the magic of crystals. This makes crystals even more effective on children and can help bring a sense of awe and wonder into their everyday lives. Practically from birth, children are able to reap the benefits of crystal healing, which can come with some bonuses. There are many crystals that can help make childbirth smoother and easier for both mother and child, and calming crystals can be used in a baby's bedroom to encourage deeper and more restful sleep. Crystals can be used to protect children from nightmares and slightly temper or encourage specific moods, and in the early stages can even be used as a healing tool. Crystals can be great for teaching children colors and shapes, and even counting. Creative little games using crystals can be thought up to stimulate their minds and creativity, all while they receive the wonderful healing energies from handling and being near the crystals. The time spent teaching your child about crystals and playing these little games with them can be a great opportunity to bond with them and develop a good relationship. In less severe situations like light colds or very minor injuries, crystals can be a much more natural alternative to chemical-based remedies. Specific crystals can also be a good way to better manage restlessness and ADD in children. A little later in life, crystals can be a great help for children at school. Having a healing crystal with them at school can children stay focused on their work, improve their skills at making friends, protect them from too much negative energy, and give them a sense of comfort and security. Especially on the first day of school or during important events, the familiar feel of a crystal lying coolly in the palm of their hand can do a lot to help your child ease off some anxiety and feel more reassured and confident.

There are some minor risks involved with introducing children to crystals. Smaller crystals can be a choking hazard for very young children, and sharp points and hard edges can hurt your child. Crystals should be kept far out of the reach of children, and it is advised to start off with round or tumbled crystals that don't have any cutting or poking edges and corners. It is also important to ensure that children aren't allowed to handle crystals without the supervision of a responsible adult until they have proven themselves to be careful and responsible enough to work with crystals on their own.

Crystal Healing for Pets

Just like with children, animals experience the same benefits from crystals. Kind words and a few crystals can help animals heal a lot faster, and their moods and behavior can be managed a little easier.

Using crystal healing on animals is a very intuitive process, as they can't communicate their problems as effectively as people, and you usually have to observe the animal and guess whether the crystal is having the right effect or not, but it becomes easier the more you spend time learning how your pet reacts. Crystals can be used to help heal illnesses and minor injuries, ease aches and pains in older animals and, in a worst-case scenario, help ease the passing of a beloved pet when it reaches the end of its life. As always, crystal healing works through proximity and contact, but it can be a little tricky to get a pet to carry one around with them. A good way to ensure a pet always has a crystal with them is to attach it to their collar. Sewing crystals into favorite toys or placing them around their favorite sleeping spots are another way to ensure that pets spend a lot of time near healing crystals. For birds and hamsters, it's a good idea to attach crystals to the outside of their cages. Many of the common techniques of crystal healing such as crystal massages and water infusions, which will be discussed in detail in the next chapter, are effective for pets too. In many cases, such as with a massage, pets will even enjoy the healing process a lot.

Chapter 6: The Science Behind Crystals

Is there any scientific proof that the crystals operate? It is an undisputed reality that quartz crystal has characteristics such as piezoelectricity, whereby its six ends alternate a favorable and negative charge under certain circumstances. And we understand that quartz can garner vast quantities of information and that crystals are used in everything from watches to computer chips to vehicles. Thanks to quantum physics, science now recognizes what the metaphysicists have been stating all along, that everything is energy, that energy can be transmuted and altered and that everything vibrates. It is also recognized that minerals don't need to be specifically ingested to be efficient and that healing is feasible throughout moment and space.

Historically, populations such as the Romans, the Ancient Egyptians, the Chinese, the Ancient Greeks, the Indians and the Ancient Japanese have used crystals to encourage relaxation, enlightenment and the appeal and satisfaction of all types of longing. The use of crystal dates back at least 6,000 years to the moment of the ancestral Sumerians of Mesopotamia. They are regarded to have metaphysical characteristics and some even assert psychic abilities periodically. So this contributes to the question, what's so unique about crystals?

All crystals (or, to be accurate, crystalline silica) is regarded to be one of the construction blocks of existence. They are produced of the two most common components on the planet—Silicon and Oxygen. The atoms bond together under stress, after which they form, extremely stably, into a three-dimensional model of repetition, providing the' crystal' its shape.

Silicon and oxygen together make up around 75% of the Earth surface. Silicon is also remarkable conductor of electricity and therefore crystals are of great use in the technology sector. These characteristics have rendered Crystalline Silica an indispensable element of the natural and technological worlds.

The glass–Quartz–is among the most secure glass buildings around and is therefore commonly used. It is widely used in transistors, in the universe of integrated circuits and is the cornerstone of all computer chips. It is utilized, as well, in all types of electronics, including phones, portable army radios and sophisticated electronic devices. In the sector of laser optics, this gem is used in the form of prisms and optical filters for timing devices. Certain crystals are also used for quartz watches and other similar equipments.

It seems that we are highly dependent on crystal technology in our daily life!

Of course, quartz is also an element of all types of land, dirt and sand. It is common in igneous, sedimentary and metamorphic stone formations. Certain microorganisms (radiolars) use a compound removed from water to create their buildings and shells. Quartz is also essential for craftsmanship in buildings. It is made of concrete and cement, as well as plastic, rubber and paint! Stone is between 70 and 90 percent quartz.

So, how do crystals function?

Quartz crystals have a very distinctive property called piezoelectricity. Mechanical stress is converted into electricity by a piezoelectric crystal. This implies that twisting or squeezing or compressing a crystal produces an electrical energy. The opposite is true as well; the electricity leads the crystal to flex, boost, or compress.

When a quartz crystal is ripped or smacked, the tension applied to it provokes an electrical charge. Once the electrical charge is transferred to the quartz, the crystal is distorted and when the voltage is withdrawn, the crystal generates an electrical field. It vibrates—sometimes 30,000 times a second! Considering that our bodies constantly produce energy, the relationship between us and the crystals is quite evident.

They also indicated that they have managed to collect vast amounts of information for more than a million years! Furthermore, the crystal was capable of thermal stability up to 1000.

Have a look at the technical spiel below if you dare.

"The prototype is made of a square of quartz two centimeters wide and two millimeters thick. It houses four layers of dots that are created with a second laser, which produces extremely short pulses of light. The dots represent information in binary form, a standard that should be comprehensible even in the distant future and can be read with a basic optical microscope. Because the layers are embedded, surface erosion would not affect them."

—From the Scientific American Journal

This report implies that crystals (specifically quartz) can stock information through laser technology (which are effective wavelengths of energy). Moreover, it suggests that this mechanism works notably well with high-intensity fluctuations. This is especially beneficial in what concerns the absorption of other high-intensity electromagnetic waves like ionizing and non-ionizing radiation! Specific emission types (as sound, heat, sunlight) move at a lower speed and are not fully penetrating the body (non-ionizing), while other forms of radiation are faster-moving and extremely harmful (ionizing), which is the case of MRI scans and Gamma radiation. In these situations, the question is: do crystals have any properties that could be successfully used to lower the level of radiation?

The damaging effects of high intensity ionizing radiation appear to be at the core of our minds. The impact of radiation poisoning resulting from the bombing of Hiroshima and Nagasaki in 1945, for instance, can still be seen today. Nowadays, around 500 nuclear stations produce electricity around the Globe (only 10% of the total power). Following the Tsunami of 2004, a nuclear power station in Fukushima collapsed, resulting in almost one thousand tons of radioactive material discharged every day ever since into the Pacific Ocean! Subsequently, the devastating effects on underwater wildlife are alarming apparent. Could crystals maybe help to purify radiation poisoning within the oceans and absorb the high-intensity Gamma waves?

USING CRYSTALS AT NIGHT

Speaking of bedrooms, this is the perfect place for crystals, because they can assist us while we're sleeping. If we're in a dream-state, we can be more receptive to them, because our logical mind is switched off.

If you suffer from sleeping disorders, attempt putting a Selenite Tower on your bedside table, selenite is a fiber optic that captures the light and reflects it into the room. It produces a quiet room to assist with healthy sleep.

If you're keen in investigating your dreams, receiving texts through your dreams, or making a lucid dream, an attempt is putting a Labradorite rock under your pillow.

If you experience nightmares or dread during sleep, place Chrysoprase under the pillow or your bed.

You can also position four pieces of selenite, hematite or crystals in each corner of your room, creating a safety screen.

If I've had an emotional week, I'm going to sleep on rose quartz and it's not unusual to discover that I'm still carrying it when I wake up. Agates are also excellent crystals to keep while sleeping. Any rock that feels pleasant to hold on to it can assist you sleep easier.

Also for sleeping difficulties, attempt putting a grounding rock at the bottom of your bed like a Garnet, black tourmaline or a Jasper.

Finally, to help with detox during your sleep, attempt a bit of ocean jasper under your pillow or your bed. Make sure that it is rinsed and recharged with 20 minutes of sunlight every week or so.

These techniques are all cumulative. Luckily, there's not much you have to do, other than positioning the rocks, be receptive to them and let them get to work.

Remember that this is a vigorous exchange, which implies that you can take care of your rocks by maintaining them smooth, by loading them on your altar from moment to moment, or by burning a candle and putting them around it. The highest findings come when you remember to create room for appreciation every day.

Chapter 7: The Basics Of Healing Through Crystals

Now, we have come to the fifth step in achieving success in crystal healing which is the part wherein it is already necessary for us to learn the basic procedures on how to do it. Crystal healing requires presence of mind and articulation so you must be able to accomplish these things and be ready first before you perform the procedures.

The first thing that we need to learn in doing crystal healing is the concept of the chakra. The word chakra is the Sanskrit term for wheel. Chakra basically means the wheel of energy present in our bodies that perpetually revolves and rotates as long as we continue to be living entities. Chakras are not visible using the naked eye but some gifted individuals, who are called psychic, can see them. Most psychics depict chakras as colorful flowers or colorful wheels that have a core. A person's chakra runs from the base of the spinal cord up to the top of his or her head. It is located at both the front and the back of a person's body.

There are seven different chakras for the different parts of the body and these chakras rotate at different speeds. The slowest rotating chakra is the first chakra or what is commonly known as the root chakra while the fastest rotating chakra is the seventh chakra, also known as the crown chakra.

Before we go to the procedures, we must be able to locate the chakras in our bodies first. The **first chakra** or **the root chakra** is located at the base of the spine near at the tail bone at the back part and the pubic bone in the front. This is the center for one's survival, security, safety and basic needs.

The **second chakra** or **the sacral** or **belly chakra** is rooted on the spine and is situated just a few inches below the navel. It is the center for a person's sexuality, intuition, self-worth and creativity.

The **third chakra**, which is also called as **the solar plexus** is located at the center behind the stomach and a few inches away from the breast. It is the dwelling place of the ego and the center of a person's anger, personal power, strengths and impulses.

The **fourth chakra** or **the heart chakra** is where spirituality, love and compassion reside. It is located at center location between the shoulder blades at the back and behind the breast bone at the front.

The **fifth chakra** or **the throat chakra** is the center for communication, sound and the expression of thoughts and ideas. It is located at the part that resembles a letter V in the clavicles at the lower neck.

The **sixth chakra** or what is commonly known as **the third eye** is the chakra responsible for higher intuition, psychic ability, as well as the energies surrounding the light and the spirit. It can also be used in the eradication of selfishness and the purification of negative attitudes. It can be located on top of the eyes at the midpoint of the forehead.

The last and **seventh chakra** is also called **the crown chakra**. It is responsible for spirituality, powerful thought, energy, cosmic consciousness, wisdom and enlightenment. It is located at the behind the pinnacle of the skull.

Now that we have come to know the different chakras and what they are responsible for, let us now get into the procedure of crystal healing.

Crystal healing can be simply done by aligning the crystals on the specific locations where you think the chakras are affected. For example, if you have a problem with your digestive system, you just have to place a kind of crystal on the location of the belly chakra or the second chakra. That is why it is a requisite to know the location of the chakras and the kinds of crystals that they are affiliated with so that you will know where to put the right kind of crystal in order to alleviate one's symptoms and sickness.

So basically, there are five major steps in crystal healing. First is of course to diagnose what kind of sickness the person is experiencing. Next, choose and select a crystal that can best heal the person and his or her sickness, depending on the diagnosis. The third step is cleansing the crystal. The fourth step is be dedicated and attuned to the crystal that you chose. And the last but definitely not the last, is to activate, program and charge your crystal.

Why is there a need to cleanse your crystal? Well, sometimes a crystal loses its connection with you and your chakras. The crystal that you were previously comfortable with may not be as comfortable as it was now. Also when you buy a specific crystal, you never know what kind of energy is in it. Sometimes crystals have build up of negative energy that can be harmful for you instead of being beneficial. That is why you need to cleanse your crystals before you use them – so that they can be pure and ready for your usage. There are several ways on how you can cleanse your crystal. The simplest way is through clear the crystals using detergent. What you should do is clean your crystals with the detergent and then after, immerse the crystals in water until the soap bubbles disappear. You can just also run the crystals under the faucet and let the running water get rid of the soap instead of immersing them. Then after the crystals are clean, you can dry them off using a soft fabric or tablecloth.

Another way of cleansing your crystal is through smudging, which is the process of applying the smudge from the burnt cedar or sage on the crystal. There is also this unique way of cleansing crystal which is done through the process called moonlight. It is the process of exposing your crystals under the light of the full moon and letting the soft rays of the night's illumination purify the crystals.

Once you have already cleansed your crystal, the next step that you need to do is to program it. The procedure of programming a crystal is pretty easy. All you have to do is summon all the positive energy that you have and the positive energy that you can get from the world around you and then direct all of these energy into the crystal. Is just like basically transferring the positive energy that you have in your body into your crystal so that it will be filled with nothing but positivity. There are also different ways on how you can program your crystals. Some do this by just putting the crystal on their palm for a couple of minutes. Some healers also use chants, incantations and mantras in order to transfer the energy towards the crystal. Some also use a combination of these methods. They keep the crystals in their closed fists and then say an incantation or sing a chant as they close their eyes and focus their energy outwards and let it flow to the crystal.

We already know the simple way of healing through the use of crystals. The next question is: What are the ailments that it can cure? The next chapter will discuss about this.

Chapter 8: Crystal Healing Techniques

There are many ways to use crystals in healing for self and others. The simplest way to use crystals is to just have them around you. It is as simple as wearing the crystal on a ring or on a chain around your neck. There are other techniques and exercises that exist to improve the healing properties of the crystal. Some of these techniques will be discussed in this chapter.

Crystal Pendulum

Crystal pendulums are used to remove any imbalances in the body. The crystal pendulum can be of any crystal depending on the type of healing. While quartz is used for an overall healing, other crystals can be used for healing specific parts of the body.

There are a series of steps to follow for the healing to work.

➤First, the patient has to lie down with the healer seated next to them.

➤The healer should hold the pendulum between their forefinger and thumb. The pendulum should be positioned just below the feet at the central axis of the body. The pendulum should be suspended a few centimeters above the body.

➤Then, the pendulum should be swung to and fro in a slow motion. This is the neutral swing.

➤The swinging pendulum should then be moved gradually along the central axis of the body from the feet towards the head.

➤At the points of energy imbalance, the pendulum will swing away from the neutral swing. At such points, wait until the swing returns to the neutral position.

➤Repeat the process from feet to head along each side of the body. It is necessary for both the healer and patient to remain calm and relaxed throughout the entire procedure.

Crystal Wand

Crystal wands are shaped in such a way so that one end is pointed while the other is flat and smooth. These are traditionally used by healers and are seen in various sizes. The shape is important because it helps in focusing the energy into a straight line. The smooth end also helps in effective massage to relax the body.

Crystal wands can be used to rid the body of any negative energy or emotions.

There are specific steps to follow while healing with a crystal wand.

➤First, the patient has to lie down with the healer seated next to them.

➤To help the patient to relax, the smooth side of the wand can be used on the tensed spots to release the tension. The smooth end is moved in small circles over the tensed area.

➢To help with healing, begin at the feet.

➢The wand is held with its pointed head pointing outwards and rotated anticlockwise.

➢The wand is moved up the body slowly.

➢In certain parts of the body, the wand will feel heavier or there will a pull towards a particular direction. Follow the force and change the motion and return back to the normal motion in a few minutes.

➢When the wand reaches the head, reverse the position of the wand so that the pointed end faces inside. Now, move the wand downwards back to the feet. This time, move the wand in small clockwise circles, which to recharge the energy fields.

Make sure that the patient is truly relaxed before attempting the healing or it will not be effective. Spend a few extra minutes on the massaging at the starting if the patient is too tense.

Sacred Eights

Sacred Eights are used to balance the excess electromagnetic frequencies in the body. They can also be used to restore balance in the working of organs. If you have a problem with an organ, sacred eights can be used to restore their functions. Sacred eights can be used either in correlation with the chakras or for a specific organ.

While focusing on the chakras, the patient is made to lie down and relax. Then, a crystal is placed on each chakra point. Then each crystal is moved in the shape of an eight. Alternatively, the crystals can be placed to form the loop of an eight around the person.

Depending on the organ, a different type of crystal can be used. The crystal will have to be spun around the area to be healed in a loop of eight. The clarity of thought will return almost immediately after this type of healing. It helps the organ return to balance when the crystals are spun to form loops of eight. They can be used over eyes to help with vision problems and exhaustion.

The theory behind this is that one loop is considered to contain Yin energy and the other contains Yang energy. So when the 8 loop is made, the two halves of the loop coincide equally signifying a unity between Yin and Yang energy. Thus, the loop of eight leads to an energy balance in the body.

Sitting and Holding Crystals

The simplest way to use crystals is to hold a crystal that is chosen for the purpose of healing. Intuition plays a major role in the choice of crystal.

You can either hold the stone for ten to twenty minutes or you can also sit with the chosen crystals surrounding you to form a healing layout.

You can repeat this multiple times in a day.

Quartz crystal points can be used to direct energy either toward or away from a body depending on where the point is facing.

Meridian Lines

Another effective technique in crystal healing is to trace the meridian lines with crystals while stopping at acupuncture points. This method is easier when performed by somebody else.

Any example of meridian line is one that starts at the pubic bone and ends just below the lips. A crystal can be moved along this line. It will help in balancing the conception channel. People who are familiar with acupuncture can use the point to heal with crystals instead of needles.

Ao Circuit

This technique follows the path of energy centers that have been used in ancient Hawaiian traditions. It helps in improving the spiritual, mental, and emotional state of a person. It helps maintain harmony.

It has a specific procedure that goes as follows:

➢The patient is made to lie down with the healer next to them.

➢A crystal is held above the crown for a few minutes. The crown is the center of will power.

➢The crystal is then moved to the right eye.

➢From there to the right shoulder. This is the center of new beginnings.

➢The crystal is then moved to the point where the hip bone joins the right leg. This is the point of action.

➢Then to the pubic bone which is the center of anchoring.

➢ Then move the crystal to the left hip that is the center of contemplation.

➢ Then in the circuit is the right shoulder. This is the point of appreciation.

➢ The crystal is then moved to the right eye that balances the quality of justice.

➢ The last stop is the heart that signifies love.

➢ The crystal is then moved back to the crown and circled around the whole body four times.

Seated Treatment

This step ensures that the body is balanced at each chakra point. It helps in maintaining a balance with each point of the chakra and creating a harmony of energy.

➢ The patient is made to sit with the healer standing next to them.

➢The healer holds a receptive crystal in their left hand that is positioned at the back of the patient's head.

➢The projecting crystal is held in the right hand in front of the patient's head.

➢These two crystals are moved downwards to each chakra.

➢At each chakra point they are to be moved in and out in order to stimulate and balance the point.

This can be done with any type of crystal. Many people prefer to use a clear crystal as the projector and a cloudy one as the receptive crystal.

✓ The no name technique

This healing technique doesn't have a particular name. It involves two people, a healer and a patient. The healer holds a pointed crystal in their right hand and points the pointy-head towards the patient's left foot. Similarly, the crystal in the left hand points to the patient's right foot. This allows the energy to flow from the right hand of the healer to the left hand of the healer through the body of the patient.

This forms a continuous circle of energy flowing in and out. All the blocks are broken up and the unwanted, negative energies are washed away and replaced with positive energies from the crystals.

✓ You can also hold a crystal in each hand.

A clear crystal in your dominant hand to use over your body and another crystal in your other hand that acts as the receptive crystal. The latter is a crystal whose properties you want to promote in yourself.

The crystal in your dominant hand is moved from top to down following the energy fields. The crystal can also be moved in small circles.

Beside these techniques, crystals can be used in other forms to cleanse not only the body but also the atmosphere in a room. **Gemstone trees** are one such object. They are tree like structures made of crystals and other healing stones. They can be kept in a room to help clear out the negative energy.

Crystal Points are similar to wand but lack a smooth end. These are used to either remove or send energy to the body. When the crystal is pointed towards the body, it channels the energy into the body. When it is faced away, the energy is removed from the body.

Crystal Pyramids can be used to focus energy at the apex of the pyramid. They are often used at the chakra points.

Crystal Wind Chimes are made by hanging crystals from a string. These crystals, which will move when wind blows against them, are said to disperse negative energy in the atmosphere.

Sun catchers are to be hanged in a place where light will pass through. When light passes through the crystals, it will bounce around the room. It is considered to bring prosperity and good luck to the home.

Crystals can also be used to heal oneself by prolong contact.

Crystals can be worn as **accessories**. They can be worn in rings, chains, or bracelets to ensure prolonged contact with the body and hence continuous healing. The accessory can be modified depending on which part of the body is to be healed.

Crystals can also be used in the **bath**. Crystals can be placed in the water or around the bathtub. This gives a calming effect especially after a long tiring day. It helps in stress relief and removes all negative thoughts and feelings.

Gem essences are another way to heal oneself using crystals. Gem essences are liquid forms of crystal. They have the same intensity as an actual crystal. It has quicker healing properties because water is one the constituents used to make the essence. Gem essence is a mixture of water, crystal, and brandy. The crystal is soaked in an exact amount of spring water. Then take a bottle half filled with brandy. Add the soaked spring water to the bottle and shake. This is considered to be the mother essence. A drop of this mother essence is added to a bottle of water to form a gem essence. This essence can be consumed from time to time. Frequent consumption of this essence could lead to imbalance. However, the balance of water, brandy, and crystal has to be exactly right or it could become toxic.

Just keep the crystals close! Well, this is the easiest thing to do and it does not require any effort whatsoever. A crystal is a fully charged fragment of the earth and the energy given off by this will keep you going throughout the day. You can incorporate these crystals into your everyday accessories so that you can always wear them. For instance, you can incorporate it into your belt, jewelry, or even just carry it around in your pocket. But if you don't mind putting in some effort, then the alternative available to this is the practice of crystal meditation. All you need to do is place a bunch of crystals on your body and lay down. Free your body of all thoughts and relax for an hour or so, and you are bound to feel rejuvenated afterwards.

The chakra bed-Each chakra present in your body corresponds with a different crystal. Before you go to sleep, take 7 crystals, pone crystal for each chakra and place them under the mattress in the spot where you usually sleep. Throughout the duration of your sleep, the energy will be continually be transmitted into your body and absorbed by it, so that when you wake up in the morning you will feel refreshed and energetic. Many have found this method to be quite effective. Why don't you give it a whirl too, the results might pleasantly surprise you.

Spread the Love!! There is a popular African phrase that goes a follows "how can one of us be happy, if all of us are not? We are all one." This step is all about realizing the well-being of people around you. The amount of pain and suffering present in this world is just increasing by the minute. You are not only aware of this, but you also have the power to do something to change this miserable state of affairs. You can actually make a positive change in someone else's life in a very simple manner. Why don't you tuck away a crystal into your friends purse or bag, or gift someone a piece of jewelry made of crystals, you can see the ripples of positive energy generated through these crystals. In the end, all this positive energy will eventually have a positive effect on your life, too. If you happen to be a part of everything good and are also able to reduce someone else's suffering, then this transformation will heal you.

Gem Water is similar to essence, however, only water is used. The crystal is soaked in spring water overnight. It is the easiest form. It can be drunk like how water is drunk and has no adverse effects on the body. Leave some crystals to rest in water for a long period of time. Such water, for a lack of a better word, is spirit water. Take a pitcher of water and let the crystals just soak in it for a night, if not for a few hours before you consume it. The energy radiating off these crystals will be infused into the water and the structure of the water will align in a manner similar to the vibrations given by the crystals. Try this once, and it is highly likely that you might not want to drink coffee ever again; the energy radiated by it is such.

Crystals can also be placed **under a pillow**. This helps not only in healing of the body but also prevents nightmares and wards off unnecessary thoughts. It also helps overcome insomnia.

In this chapter we examined the different ways that crystals facilitate the process of healing in your body. But before we begin, you should keep in mind this golden rule. Before you start using your crystals you should place them under the sun for several hours so that they will get charged with all the positive life bearing energy radiating from the sun and this energy can be transmitted into your body.

Chapter 9: Crystals- So Pretty And Helpful To Us

As the earth was shaped, gems were made. They originate from a bounty of minerals found in the world's surface. Substance debasements, sand and sun-powered discharges, and radiation have created a variety of precious stones with various hues, shapes, and energies.

Precious stones have been utilized to help mend, stimulate, or quiet the piece of the body that requirements are adjusting. They do this by vibrating or attracting energies to you. Here are a few gems and their forces.

Agate precious stones come in various hues; blue-green, green, pink, and blue trim which is light blue with white or darker lines. They have fantastic defensive and mending energies. They draw in riches and wellbeing, and they are the best mending stones. They help with issues of the teeth and gums. They help the circulatory system, colon, heartbeats, and pancreas.

The precious stone Amethyst is purple. It is the stone of profoundly and satisfaction. It is useful for contemplation and reinforcing the clairvoyant capacities. Amethyst quiets the brain and disintegrates uneasiness. It helps with recuperating addictions of assorted types and disciplined practices.

Sea green/blue is a light blue shading. It quiets the nerves, gives mental clarity, helps fears and fears, and equalizations feelings. It is useful for the eyes and sight.

Citrine is a light orange shading. It assists with self-articulation and advances fearlessness, and It changes negative energy to positive. It's known as the dealer's stone since it pulls in cash and new business and improves sales.

Peridot is a light green shading. It is a passionate healer and pardoning stone. It helps balance your feelings, discharges negative vibrations, and advances prosperity. It is likewise a cash stone.

There is clear and shake precious stone quartz. Quartz is an ace recuperating stone. It amplifies the energies of different precious stones. Negative power will be fended off. Clear quartz draws energy to you.

Red quartz is a ruddy shading. It expands energy levels, memory review, and makes positive activity. It reinforces red platelets and helps blood course.

Rose quartz is a light pink stone. It is known as the heart stone. Wear or convey this to attract love to you, make love among you and somebody extraordinary, and to mend a messed up heart. It fortifies the heart and circulatory systems, supporting chest and lung issues.

Rutilated quartz can be drab or smoky with brilliant dark-colored, dark, or ruddy strands. It helps simplicity fears and depression. Gets the energy moving on all levels. Moderates the maturing procedure and assists with mental focus.

Smoky quartz has a tarnish to blackish tint, in some cases yellowish. It's a tremendous defensive stone that helps stop negative energies. It's useful with gloom and weariness.

Tigers Eye quartz is green with whorls of dark experiencing it. It draws in riches. Mellows determination. Helps your fearlessness and internal quality. Helps your stomach, processing, ulcers, and skeletal structure.

After you purchase precious stones and before you wear them they must be absorbed saltwater overnight after you wear them for a moment, you'll need to drench them again to re-energize them. Envelop your precious stones by a delicate fabric when you're not wearing them to ensure them. The gems that give you energy shouldn't be worn around evening time.

When the gems have been doused, you should devote them to the reason for which you use them. The precious stones will draw on that particular energy. Hold the precious stone and think about the specific purpose for which you need to utilize it. State for all to hear "I program this gem for (your motivation). You might need to rehash this multiple times, and after each time you douse them.

You could ruminate with your gem. Grasp it and inhale delicately. As you inhale out, let go of any pressure and as you take in, let harmony stream in. Take a gander at your precious stone and notice it's shading and shape. Feel it's vibrations. At that point, close your eyes and consider the energy of the precious stone. Whenever done, open your eyes and put the precious stone down.

Crystal Healing - Unblocks The Negative Patterns

Precious stone recuperating, as a treatment in it, might seem, by all accounts, to be new, utilizing thoughts and strategies from numerous societies joined together; however, the present-day enthusiasm for gem mending is a continuation of humanity's interest with gemstones and minerals down the ages.

Gem mending unblocks the negative examples by raising the vibrational recurrence of the energy field that encompasses your body. Since recuperating is the way toward working with the energy handle that comprises your body, with the assistance of gems you will have included essentialness and feel like everything is ok once more.

The energy field is the energy of the spirit.

Working with the energy of the spirit is the most elevated type of mediation you can get. Since it is the most productive approach to distinguish and kill the main drivers of both mental and physical ailment. Gems do this by taking a shot at the body energy centers, known as the 'Chakras.' At the point when the 'Chakras ' are not working effectively, you will feel unwell or tied.

Precious stone recuperating in some structure or another has been rehearsed by pretty much every general public on earth, a considerable lot of which had profoundly established conviction frameworks that bolstered comprehensive thoughts and strategies. Without this social foundation, precious stone mending has, to a great extent, turned into a territory of confidence and "flakiness." You either "accept" gems can mend, or you don't, with practically zero levelheaded clarification of how it may function

These precious stones were ground up and sprinkled legitimately on wounds, and researcher today have demonstrated that it is a potent bactericide. Others accept gem mending is even more seasoned, starting in the old human progress of Atlantis or conceivably even ' Lemuria.' The ancient Greek and Roman healers, for example, Pliny and Galen utilized Hematite for cerebral pains. Pliny likewise used it for blood issue. In any case, the one common conviction was the enormous potential of recuperating properties that these stones contained.

Herbal Remedies for Urinary Tract Infections - How You Can Use Remedies Found at Home to Treat a UTI

Is it true that you are a lady who continually battles with agonizing UTI's? It is safe to say that you are finished inclination along these lines, and do you wish that you could feel much improved? If you are wary of managing the consistent torment and with the consuming sensation, at that point, you need some assistance.

Presently isn't an ideal opportunity to race to the specialist's so the individual can review you a costly remedy. Indeed, even idea that may feel like the most straightforward arrangement right now, it will wind up costing you more cash than it ought to, and you could conceivably get the help that you are searching for. When you hope to dispose of your UTI and quick, at that point, it's time that you took care of business and that you assumed responsibility for your wellbeing.

You are searching for specific ways that can assist you with getting the alleviation that you are searching for in a characteristic, shoddy, and safe way. You would prefer not to be compelled to go to the specialist's and fortunately, you don't need to. You can dispose of your urinary tract contamination all from the solace of your home and by utilizing common home cures.

There are numerous natural solutions for urinary tract diseases, and they all can work for you. They are general, and they help ladies to get the alleviation from the torment and the consuming.

An incredible cure that you should attempt above all else is for you to drink; however, much fluid during your time as could be expected. You have to drink many liquids since you have to continue peeing. Although ousting pee is exceptionally disturbing, you have to do it since you have to keep the contamination moving out of you. The more you pee, the more the microscopic organisms will be removed from your body. Peeing that discharge out of your body harms yet is gainful to your body. Take a stab at including some lemon for taste, yet for treatment also. Adding lemon to your water can free your body of those poisons and microorganisms considerably quicker.

Another homegrown solution for your urinary tract disease is to kill the corrosive in your pee since that will facilitate a portion of the torment. The ideal approach to execute a caustic is to utilize an essential power against it. The best thing to use is the heating soft drink. Take a stab at blending some heating soft drink with some water and drinking it. It will flush through your body, an assault that microorganisms, help to kill the corrosive in your pee, and make utilizing the washroom somewhat simpler.

You don't need to feel defenseless in regards to your UTI any longer. If you utilize these means likewise and utilize these medicines, you will most likely get alleviation, and you will probably feel preferred a lot quicker over with physician recommended meds.

Herbal Remedies for Psoriasis 4 Highly Useful Remedies

Psoriasis is brought about by the development of abundance skin cells; it's not irresistible so it can't be moved. It is an autoimmune ailment, so treating it might be intense. Discovering great herbal solutions for psoriasis may lighten the redness and irritation. Continue perusing to see which ones are better.

Psoriasis isn't in every case, simple to analyze. However, there are five essential kinds of psoriasis. They are reverse, plaque, guttate, pustular, and endothermic psoriasis. Some primary side effects of psoriasis are dry, irritated skin, gleaming plaque development, little stick point draining, and layered skin. In any case, when you make sense of that you have psoriasis there probably won't be any prescription promptly accessible to you. Here are four lesser-known cures of psoriasis than can take care of business, and in particular they aren't unreasonably costly.

Shark Cartilage: This is an enhancement produced using the dried and powdered ligament of sharks. This enhancement has gigantic anti-inflammatory properties, which are valuable when treating psoriasis.

Night Primrose Oil: Research demonstrates that this oil helps treat psoriasis since it adds gamma-linolenic corrosive to the client. This vital unsaturated fat common is in limited quantities in people living with psoriasis.

Milk Thistle: This herbal solution for psoriasis assists with the generation of T Cells and like this incredibly accommodating when attempting to treat psoriasis.

Oregano: This natural family unit herb is anything but complicated to drop by and with its antibacterial and antifungal properties, it is advantageous with helping psoriasis. These general properties help to keep diseases from framing in the psoriasis plaques.

Home Remedies For Sweaty Palms - Useful Remedy to Cure Excessive Hand Sweating

Sweaty palms are humiliating since they influence your own life seriously, yet also public activity. Envision that some odder is happy to meet you and stretches out his hand to shake your hand. Right now, if the outsider contacted your sweaty hand, at that point envision how it will humiliate for you and clumsy for the outsider. In this circumstance, you need to fix your sweaty palms promptly. Sweaty palms isn't a dangerous condition. However, it is unusual, since your hands sweat exorbitantly when the others don't sweat by any stretch of the imagination. In any case, some valuable home cures can fix your inordinate hand perspiring.

It is your eating routine that can influence your perspiring straightforwardly. Iodine is the critical component that triggers your perspiration organs to actuate. In this way, chop down the admission of nourishment that incorporates iodine. Abstain from taking salt in an excessive sum. Other than this, you ought to likewise stay away from white onions, broccoli, asparagus, hamburger, liver, turkey, and so on. Drinking sage tea proves an effective home cure over the sweaty palms. You can likewise attempt a tea arrangement as a home solution for sweaty hands. Douse your hands into the tea answer for 15-20 minutes by the day's end, before you head to sleep. It is the tannic corrosive of the tea arrangement that causes effectively to diminish gentle perspiring.

Most importantly, iontophoresis is the best solution to fixing your sweaty palms. In this treatment, you have to absorb your palms two plates loaded up with water. Presently associate the gadget and keep your palms in the dish for 20 minutes. Rehash this session on a consistent schedule for seven days. You will find your hands evaporated. To hold the degree of dryness, you have to rehash one session thrice seven days. The market estimation of the iontophoresis machine is exceptionally high. In any case, I have built up the home iontophoresis gadget, which works effectively as like the instant one, and it is financially savvy moreover.

Presently you can fix your sweaty palms with the homemade iontophoresis machine until the end of time.

Home Remedy For Sweaty Palms - Useful Remedies to Get Rid of Excessive Hand Sweating

Many individuals have been experiencing this problem called Palmer Hyperhidrosis. Regardless of how terrible the problem is or how minute the question is, it is a humiliating one. Having sweat-soaked palms can end up being an embarrassing thing where open or get-togethers or gatherings are concerned. The vast majority abstain from shaking hands or getting stuff in dread of shame. Subsequently, this problem isn't only a physical issue yet additionally hampers yourself certainty. In such a situation, how would you take care of this problem?

There is a lot of tips accessible on the web about restoring sweat-soaked palms. If you run an inquiry, you will discover a lot of home cures on getting your palms dry once more. In any case, the majority of the occasions these are impermanent measures, and if your hyperhidrosis issue is a genuine one for you, at that point, it emerges back again in a couple of days. Subsequently, when you are one of the individuals who have been experiencing sweat-soaked palms on a positive note and for quite a while, you need a treatment called Iontophoresis. This treatment incorporates giving minute stuns to your palms to hinder the digestion rate. This electric stuns are not genuine overwhelming ones.

They are quite minute, and you scarcely feel anything. The impact is phenomenal. Presently to discover some spot which hosts Iontophoresis gear is extreme so you can locate a manual which causes you to assemble the device and develop an Iontophoresis set straight in your home. Following this treatment procedure for, at any rate, 15 minutes daily will help and get your sweat-soaked palms dry forever.

Avoid items, which guarantee to fix sweat-soaked palms effectively and in only days. Sweat-soaked palm is an old problem looked by a lot of ages, and every one of these items has neglected to convey. It is ideal to pursue the proposals which have worked for many individuals, and it is Iontophoresis.

Chapter 10: Esoteric And Evolutionary Expansion

Crystals and Sun Signs (Astrology in focus)

Since we first walked on this planet, we have looked upwards and gazed at the heavens, convinced that divine forces in the sky control our destiny. For over four thousand years, astrology has been an important influence. The seven major planets in our solar system symbolize the mixture and interaction of all essential forces of the universe and nature. This seven-fold nature of the planets also corresponds to the seven rainbow colors, and seven notes of the musical scale. Thus, throughout our lives, we have the melody of our ruling planets in our bodies and never is this planetary influence so strong as at the moment when we are born. Both mother and child need their appropriate stones near them at that time, to strengthen the planetary influences even further. Seven has always been a mystical number- it is tied in with the seven chakras and seven ages of man. So the number seven pervades our whole universe. Numerology developed as another way of showing the harmonies and relationships of the divine forces.

As we discover new planets, there being nine known planets at this time, this is in keeping with the discovery of the eighth and ninth chakras. It is believed by some that 12 planets will be found in all, relating to the twelve semitones of the chromatic scale in music. It is also possible that as

humankind evolves and raises their vibrations they will begin to see new scales of color.

There are ninety or so chemical elements that constitute all matter on earth. These are represented in the planets as well as the human body and the earth's minerals themselves. This means that we are not different and isolated from the earth or the universe. Our bodies reverberate to celestial vibrations through the medium of precious stones. Thus, precious stones can attract the planetary forces to us. When we understand this, we can use certain stones to attract to us the planetary forces that govern us at birth. These are the forces our soul needs to help it on its path in this life-time- crystals and gemstones can act as electrical receivers, receiving the electro-magnetic vibrations from its owner's planetary ruler and transmitting them with increased power. It is also useful to wear or use stones that are not astrologically matched with your planet, as we are not born under the rule of one planet alone. The forces are created by the harmonies and configurations of all the planets at the time of birth.

For each star sign there are three related stones, which shows how connected we are to the mineral kingdom as three represents the mind, body and spirit and regarding geometry and the building blocks of life; there are three sides to a triangle which is the shape from which others and the 'spiral of life' originate, which further connects all life on earth. This connection also extends to space and the cosmos itself as gem and crystal energies are established due to astrological proceedings. We can therefore establish which crystals are best used on an individual basis due to our sun sign, as we ourselves are affected by planets and celestial bodies. One gem should have high vibration energy and should be clear and bright, representing purity and love. A touchstone brings harmony, healing and peace and a talisman stone brings protection, showing how the energies of the three stones differ yet together bring balance and healing to one's life. In addition to portraying how gemstones are compatible with astrological energies, Marlene Houghton in **'An Astrological Apothecary'** suggests that one can ascertain when one is likely to become unwell or suffer specific imbalances due to the upcoming astrological alignments, therefore by being knowledgeable of one's astrological chart and the planetary energies affecting each sun sign, one can use specific gems to heal, balance and keep their electromagnetic field protected and in a state of health. Gems, henceforth, can act as preventative health care.

Over hundreds of years, the planets move in relation to the calendar, and we should not rely on calculations that were correct centuries ago. This is why conscientious astrologers will make corrections for these changes and planetary shifts. Each stone is related to the vibrations of a particular planet. This planet will also be connected to a color and a musical note. Every planet

and stone can also be linked to one of four metaphysical elements, earth, water, air and fire. Let's explore this now.

	SUN	MOON	MERCURY	VENUS	MARS	JUPITER	SATURN
COLOR	gold yellow orange	silver white	grey yellow	emerald-green	red scarlet	blue	black indigo
GEM	Topaz Diamond	Pearl Quartz	Agate Opal	Turquoise Emerald	Ruby	Amethyst Sapphire	Onyx Sapphire

The matter of color correspondences is very subjective, this is just a rough guide. They are, however, a good starting point from which to explore and experiment. They work on a deep level within your subconscious, they are not in the realm of objective reasoning. If you wish to experiment with different colors, that's fine but please make sure that you are listening to your intuitive voice within, not to your conscious mind.

Birthstones (Zodiac Astrology & Crystals)

The first step in gem healing is to make use of your birthstones. Become aware of their powers. Hold them, wear them and keep them near you. You will get to recognize their energies and connect with their spiritual consciousness. If you are treating a patient, you can also recommend they obtain three stones related to their star sign. One stone should be a precious gem. This stone should be clear and bright, bringing with it high vibrations and qualities of inspiration, purity and clarity and the highest love. The second stone should be a touchstone, one that brings you harmony, peace and healing. The third stone is a talisman, a stone of protection.

Now let us look at the Zodiac signs and the planetary forces.

Signs of the Zodiac and Color

Aries: Red stones

Taurus: Yellow and Pink stones

Gemini: Violet stones

Cancer: Green stones

Leo: Gold or orange stones

Virgo: Purple stones

Libra: Yellow stones

Scorpio: Red or crimson stones

Sagittarius: Deep blue stones

Capricorn: Black and White stones

Aquarius: Clear blue stones

Pisces: Soft blue and indigo stones

To recap, seven is an extremely significant number as it reflects mankind's connection to the universe and shows how there are recurring patterns within nature that link mankind's evolution with the cosmic vibration. The body has seven major chakras which link with the earth's major chakra points, and just like the body has meridians and energy zones- our planet has lay lines and energy grids. One can connect to these on the energetic and auric planes to promote planetary and individual healing. The seven chakras also correspond with the seven main planets, as, in the last age of Pisces before the 2012 equinox, there were only seven major planets recorded; however now as this cycle is an octave up on a higher and more unifying vibration, some sun signs have more than one planet... Pisces has the ancient and modern rulers of Jupiter and Neptune, for example. Numerology further supports 'as above so below' as pure light is split into the seven colors of the rainbow which run through our bodies, and the colors vibrate at specific frequencies relating to the chakra points, in addition to there being seven notes in the musical scale.

For a clearing treatment the client must lie with their head in a northern direction and their feet in a southern direction so they are naturally aligned to the earth's energies. One must make a six-pointed star around the client but first must create an aura of white light to protect the client from harmful energies, which is achieved by starting at the crown and walking clockwise round the client whilst visualizing and intending the white light protection. The six crystals are placed as follows: one above the crown, one crystal next to each knee, one crystal next to each elbow, and one crystal between the feet in line with the crystal above the crown. All crystals should be facing upwards as the purpose is to clear negative energy and fire energy from the sun cannot be contaminated itself, therefore the negative energy passes up through the crown without being detrimental to the surrounding environment. Once the six-pointed star has been formed a generator crystal should be used to link the crystal energies by holding the generator in both hands with the point facing downwards and passing it over the crystals six times. Once again, intentions of healing and love should be directed and visualizing white light energy linking the crystals can amplify the healing energies. It is necessary to make aware the importance of the six pointed star used in clearing treatments as it has a lot of historical, biblical and religious meaning, however with specific regards to healing it is the six pointed star that is used as a symbol for the heart or anahata chakra and represents harmony and balance, which corresponds with the intention of a crystal healing treatment.

If a client has painful or sensitive feet a crystal can be used to draw out negative energy from the feet reflexes and can be achieved by making small anti-clockwise circles with a quartz crystal. The circles should increase in size as the crystal moves away from each foot and the healer should visualize the energy being drawn out. Kirlian photography shows how our electromagnetic field or aura is actually affected by crystals and other natural healing methods such as meditation and it is through the feet that one's energy is connected to the earth's energy. Pain or sensitivities in the feet are often related to the root chakra therefore using the mentioned method on the feet can help the client become more grounded and balanced and create a freer flow of energy. The Egyptians and many ancient cultures were aware of our connection to the earth's energies through the feet and would often walk barefoot for grounding, therefore the healer could suggest this with the client and also offer suggestions such as reflexology and meditation practices to help heal and balance their root chakra. If there is a noticeable difference of energy between each foot then this will show an imbalance between the dualistic nature of energy, masculine and feminine, as it is the left brain hemisphere that affects the right hand side of the body and the right brain hemisphere that affects the left side. The right hemisphere perceives from a unifying, holistic or feminine viewpoint and the left hemisphere from an individual, egotistical and masculine perspective. Therefore, feeling which foot is over or under active will help determine the course of healing for the client and which crystals should be used as it is the mind that affects the health of the body's energy systems.

Crystal Treatments and advanced techniques

Once you have become familiar with crystals and integrated their use and application into your daily reality, you can proceed onto providing **crystal treatments**, if you should so resonate. Crystal healing treatments realign the body's energy fields, opening up the chakras to promote an overall feeling of well-being. The crystals which are placed around the body set up specific and complex electro-magnetic force fields. This energy acts to re-polarize any fields that are misaligned, redistributing the correct energies to restore harmony and balance to both the physical and subtle bodies. Physical hands are never laid directly on the body, or the healer (yourself as the channel) is at risk of picking up the negative energy from the patient. Your hands should be used to smooth out any stickiness or buildup of trapped energy in the etheric (radiating from the physical body for about 4-6 inches). The crystals correct this imbalanced energy, while your hands concentrate and direct the flow.

Preparing to Give A Crystal Treatment

Below we describe a series of treatments which should be done one after the other on the same day. Really they are stages in a single treatment. Ideally all treatments should begin with opening and balancing the chakras. Don't forget that the session should end by closing the chakras again, otherwise the client will be too open to outside negative influences. The chakras should only be open when in a safe and loving environment. If you link you can close the chakras with a visualization exercise. One by one, starting at the crown, visualize the chakra being closed, anticlockwise, like a camera lens iris. Make sure you have a quiet, warm, and comfortable place for the treatment, and make sure that you will not be disturbed.

Remove any electrical equipment from the room, as these interfere with the magnetic fields even if they are switched off. Ask your client or friend to remove any metal objects, watch, jewelry, belts or coins. Also make sure they are wearing comfortable loose clothing. Your client might like to bathe before a crystal treatment. It is most common to get the client to lie on their back initially, so they can see what you are doing if they wish to do so. You may however, wish to work on the back during the treatment, in which case they will have to turn face down. Always explain to them what you are doing as they are taking an active part in their treatment.

The ideal direction for working with crystals is the north/south orientation. The reason for this is to align the body to the Earth's magnetic field and so enhance the flow of the crystal energy. The head should point north and the feet south. In the Southern hemisphere this orientation should be reversed. We will also talk about the direction of movement. You put good energy in (infusing) by moving in a clockwise direction and you take bad energy out (clearing) in an anti-clockwise direction. What have clocks got to do with it? Absolutely nothing, but before we had clocks, we had sundials, so the shadow went around in the same direction that the sun appears (as was once thought) to go around the earth. Rather than "clockwise" it's better to think "sunwise". In other words, when working sunwise we are in harmony with the natural order of things.

However before beginning any treatment (and this is especially true in the case of clearings) it's a good idea to cast a protective circle around yourself and your client. This is to protect you both from and negative energy that may be hanging about. You don't need to make a big deal out of this. Just walk around the client clockwise (sunwise) and visualize a cone of white light surrounding you. It's a bit like an unborn chick protected inside its shell. You don't need to make a big thing out of it and your client does not even need to know you are doing it. You should reverse the procedure at the end of the treatment to open the circle before leaving.

To begin, always tune in to the client's higher self. Hold your hands above their head, and ask that they be given healing for their highest good. When you complete the treatment, give thanks for what has been received in a similar way. This is the main intention for providing any crystal treatment or clearing.

It is important to remember that a treatment will do one or a combination of the following:

CLEARING: clearing negative and blocked energy.

INSTILLING and BALANCING: replacing the negative energy with positive vibrations and strengthening and building chakra energy.

EXPANDING: for awareness and spiritual development.

Clearing Technique

Starting at the crown, walk slowly in a clockwise direction, making a circle of energy around the body, creating an auric seal, as described at the start of this lesson. You will need 6 crystal points and a generator. Place a crystal above the crown pointing upwards. Place one crystal on the outside of each knee, you are forming a triangle with the crown crystal.

Now place one crystal between the feet pointing upwards, lining it up with the crown crystal. Place the two remaining crystals at the side of the elbows. This forms a triangle with the crystal at the feet. You have formed a six-pointed star.

Now, link the energies of the crystals together holding the generator crystal in both hands with its point facing downwards. Pass the generator five more times over the crystals, then put the generator to one side. Let the client remain in this position for several minutes.

Ask them to slowly become aware of the room and then open their eyes. When they are ready, ask them for any reactions. Did they feel any difference in the new energy?

Combined Clearing and Strengthening Technique

First you need to choose stones to lay on the chakras. You may choose a stone either intuitively or you can dowse for it using a pendulum. To start with, it is useful to choose a stone which color harmonizes with the chakra. It is beneficial to lay stones in the following order: -

Choose one for - The third eye, the heart, Solar-plexus, Sacral, Crown - lay this stone above the crown, Base - lay this stone between the client's legs.

You may like to use a large clear quartz crystal over the crown, pointing downwards. For the base chakra use a stone connected to the earth energy, e.g. rose quartz or smoky quartz. The direction the clear quartz points depends on whether you are clearing or instilling the energy of the stones. If you are clearing, it should point away from the body. If you are instilling or balancing the crystal should point towards the body.

It is possible to substitute a clear quartz crystal for any stone on the layout. If a stone falls off the client during a treatment, do not touch it or replace it. It has either given the correct energy balance or it is not in tune with the client's vibrations. Once you have laid the stones on the chakras you can then use a crystal quartz to amplify the overall balance of life-energy.

Once you have placed your chakra stones, it is best to start all treatments with a simple clearing technique. Place a large clear quartz crystal above the crown chakra, pointing downwards (masculine energy) and a rose quartz or another crystal with feminine energy, between the legs pointing upwards.

Using a small clear quartz crystal in your right hand, make small harmonious circles down the left-hand side of your client, and up the right-hand side. Connect your crystal to the top and bottom crystals. Do this three times to clear the energy.

Leave the client with the chakra stone layout for 10-15 minutes. Ask them for their reactions and note it down.

Opening and Balancing the Chakras

Opening and Balancing Technique 1

You will need six crystals as in the clearing technique 2; 1 crown, 1 foot, 2 knees, 2 elbows all pointing upwards. First place 7 small crystals over each chakra all with their points up. If you wish you can choose different stones for the individual chakras. Link the outside crystals with your generator seven times, to form a protective seal.

Run the generator straight up from the feet through the chakras to the head, then down from the head to the feet. Do this five times. You can now balance the chakra energy using the palms of your hands, smoothing out any buildup of energy which you feel. Balance two chakras at a time. Try and feel the buildup of energies with your palms, you can push the energy up and down until a balance is reached.

Balance the: -

CROWN and THROAT

THIRD EYE and HEART

THROAT and SOLAR-PLEXUS

HEART and SACRAL

SOLAR-PLEXUS and BASE

You can focus more energy with your hands, or you may wish to instill or draw out energy from any chakra which you feel is under or over energized using a crystal point, in the way described for clearing or instilling energy. To instill energy into a chakra, hold the clear crystal point facing downwards, over the chakra to be balanced. Hold it in your sending hand. Now rotate the crystal in a clockwise direction. Form decreasing circles until the crystal finally touches the stone on the chakra.

You can now clear individual chakras if there is accumulated energy. Hold a clear quartz crystal in your sending hand, pointing towards the fingertips, and rotate four to twelve inches above the stone on each chakra, until each area has received enough energy.

Run your sensing hand over the etheric of the client feeling where there may be areas of stickiness or buildup of energy. Once you have felt which areas need clearing, use either a clear quartz crystal or a stone relating to the area needing clearing. Holding your receiving hand over the chakra, and a crystal, point facing downwards, in your sending hand out to one side of you. Now rotate the crystal anti-clockwise down by your side. You are using yourself as a transmitter, lifting out the energy with your receiving hand and out through the crystal at your side.

Leave your client for a few minutes or until they are ready to focus their attention in the room. Ask them what they felt and make notes of any emotional or physical reactions. This can help you to understand energy and the power and use of crystals, and aid in any future treatments you may wish to give.

You will have first given your client a clearing and balancing treatment, and now you can begin to give them one or more building treatments. You will need 6 clear quartz crystals. Place one crystal at the crown, pointing downwards. You are instilling energy from the stones into the etheric. Place another at the feet pointing upwards. Place one at the left shoulder and one at the right shoulder, both pointing inwards. Place one at the left and one at the right knee, both pointing inwards. Connect the outer crystals in a clockwise direction to form a protective seal.

Now choose stones for each chakra, according to the type of treatment your client needs. You could dowse to see which treatment is needed.

You can also ask the client to visualize a safe place they can go to mentally. For instance, if this place is focused on water, they will need emotional balancing. If it is an image of sky and clouds, they will need air energy. Play gentle music which encompasses one of the four elements, while giving the gemstone treatment.

Instead of Laying Each Stone on The Chakra Directly You Can Use It to Instill Its Energy Like A Laser Beam.

To do this, hold the stone in your right hand and make clockwise circles over the chakra, in decreasing circles until you feel the chakra has received enough energy. This is sending concentrated energy into the chakra. You may need to diffuse some of this energy, and to do this form circles anti-clockwise, spreading the energy over a wider area.

Earth, Air, Fire & Water...

Here are some specific crystals you can use for unique effects.

GROUNDING (earth)

Root: Garnet

Sacral: Cornelian

Solar-plexus: Chrysoprase

Heart: Jade

Throat Blue: Lace Agate

Third Eye: Sodalite

Crown: Blue Kyanite

NEW BEGINNINGS (earth)

Root: Bloodstone

Sacral: Rhodonite

Solar-plexus Green Tourmaline/chalcedony

Heart: Rhodochrosite

Throat: Celestite

Third Eye: Blue sapphire/turquoise

Crown: Clear quartz

EMOTIONAL BALANCE (water)

Root: Smoky quartz

Sacral: Aventurine

Solar-plexus: Green Tourmaline

Heart: Rose quartz

Throat: Aquamarine

Third: Blue sapphire/moonstone

Crown: Clear quartz

RELEASING THE PAST (water)

Root: Black tourmalinated quartz

Sacral: Watermelon tourmaline

Solar-plexus: Green tourmaline

Heart: Pink Tourmaline

Throat: Aquamarine

Third Eye: Moonstone

Crown: Clear quartz

MANIFESTING YOUR WISDOM (air)

Root: Tiger's eye

Sacral: Orange cornelian

Solar-plexus: Blue Tourmaline/ Jade

Heart: Peridot

Throat: Aquamarine

Third Eye: Yellow Topaz/ citrine

Crown: Diamond/ clear quartz

MAKING CHANGES IN YOUR LIFE (fire)

Root: Tiger's eye

Sacral: Orange cornelian/ amber

Solar-plexus: Amber/ citrine

Heart: Ruby/ Peridot

Throat: Aquamarine/ Blue lace agate

Third Eye: Opal/ Lapis Lazuli

Crown: Amethyst/ clear quartz

Expanding Consciousness

Expanding on from the previous section of crystal treatments, here is a final layout that can be used to raise one's vibrations, connecting one to the ground and the spiritual forces. It is advisable that the client should practice a crystal meditation after this treatment as they will be receptive to higher energies.

You will need 9 crystals, 1 double terminator.

Place the double terminator above the crown.

Place a crystal between the feet.

Place a crystal on the outside of each foot, pointing outwards.

Place a crystal at each ankle also pointing outwards.

Place a crystal on each side of the neck and one at the ears.

All the crystals point outwards.

With a generator pointing downwards, link the crystal around the head starting at the left side of the neck. Move in a clockwise direction forming a FIGURE OF EIGHT crossing the body at the base chakra, and forming a circle linking the crystals around the feet. Continue to make a figure of eight six more times. Leave your client for about 15 minutes, and then remove the crystals.

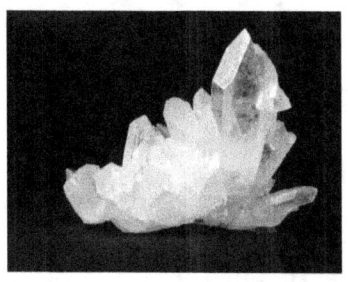

This is an extremely powerful healing arrangement and should not be used on anyone who has not had several clearing and building treatments, or at the very least has been working with crystal for a long period of time.

The 12 Zodiac Signs

If you are fascinated by crystals and their metaphysical properties you will most likely be equally intrigued by various other esoteric schools of thought. **Astrology** is primarily based on the study of the 12 signs of the zodiac. Now, as everyone reading this is one of 12 signs, we have decided to conclude this book with a section for personal self-discovery. The key to know is that choosing to learn about crystals and their uses naturally opens you up to self-evolution, and new pathways and channels for healing (wholeness, balance & integration) and self-development. Thus, learning about your **star sign** with a brief mention of the best crystals for you is the perfect way to conclude **Crystals for Beginners**.

Without further ado, here is an introduction to the 12 signs of zodiac with reference to your favored crystals.

Aries

Aries is the first sign of the zodiac and a fire sign. Symbolized by the Ram, you are fiery, bold, courageous and independent. Aries are self-starters and initiators with a highly inventive and innovative nature, you are passionate, motivated and confident, and do not suffer fools gladly! However, because of such a "head-strong" character and personality, you are often prone to impulsiveness, severe impatience, anger and short-temper verging on aggressiveness. Being ruled by planet Mars exasperates this.

In saying this, Aries is optimistic, enthusiastic and determined and can often inspire others with their sheer inner strength and passionate nature. You are at your best when channeling your energy into some creative passion-project or work pursuit. You're at your worst when giving in to "Martian" characteristics and behaviors. (Aggression, lust, war-like tendencies and extreme competitiveness!)

Best gemstones & crystals for Aries: Bloodstone, carnelian, citrine, garnet

Taurus

Taurus is an earth sign represented by the glyph, the Bull. Taurus likes security, stability and responsibility, and is reliable, patient, practical and responsible. Yet, Taurus is also highly sensual and creative, both in tune with the practical duties and responsibilities of the physical world and inner currents and feelings. This is largely due to Venus, your ruler. Venus is the planet of beauty, love, sensuality, sexuality, prosperity and luxury. Abundance and a love for the finer things in life accompany the energy of Venus, and Taurus is generally most happy when materialistically abundant and blessed. At the worst, Taurus can be stubborn, extremely rigid and inflexible, possessive and aggressive.

Some highly favored activities for Taurus sign include reading, cooking, gardening, music, romance, working outdoors or with the earth, learning and engaged in higher study or wisdom acquisition, and making love! You are a lover at heart and have a feminine energy to you, regardless of whether you're a man or a woman.

Best gemstones & crystals for Taurus: Sapphire, malachite, jade, rose quartz, pyrite, peridot

Gemini

Gemini is the Twins, another dual sign represented by the qualities of curiosity, intellect, sociability, communication, adaptability, gentleness and affection. Geminis are extremely mentally gifted and cerebral, you learn new ideas and concepts very quickly. As an air sign also ruled by the planet Mercury, Gemini excels at the arts, writing, communication and self-expression. You are fun seeking, sociable, communicative and often restless. At your worst, you can be nervous, indecisive, impractical and moody, also struggling with anxious tendencies.

Family and friendship are very important to Geminis, as are creative outlets. You are one of the most quick-witted and intelligent signs of the zodiac.

Best gemstones & crystals for Gemini: Agate, chalcedony, citrine, jade

Cancer

Cancer is a water sign with the symbol the Crab. Sensitive, moody, emotional, family-oriented and supportive, Cancers make excellent friends, support workers, counsellors, therapists, care workers, and compassionate helpers translating into charity or welfare causes. Cancers are loyal, sympathetic, empathic, imaginative, artistic, impressionable and persuasive. You possess a great understanding of emotions and can equally connect to others on an emotional level. When at your lowest, you can be pessimistic, manipulative and over-sensitive, hence the expression "withdrawing into a crab-like shell!" Cancer is ruled by the Moon and therefore is considerably in tune with the subconscious.

Favored activities include art, cooking, home-based activities, creative and imaginative self-expression, helping loved ones, music, and spending time with friends and family. You are also deeply instinctual, kind and caring.

Best gemstones & crystals for Cancer: Emerald, moonstone, citrine, red jasper, pearl

Leo

Leo is a fire sign represented by the Lion. This sign is ruled by the Sun and Leos are generally passionate, expressive, loyal, honest, fiercely protective of loved ones, creative, warm-hearted, generous and cheerful. You are a majestic creature who believes in the equal giving and receiving of love and affection. When you are in love or care for a friend or family member, your generosity and selfless nature knows no bounds! But, you also expect the same levels of love and even admiration. Your greatest downfall is excessive pride combined with a very big ego.

But, Leos have the warmest hearts and are kind, selfless and community oriented. you are also incredibly passionate with a strong creative nature and life force.

Best gemstones & crystals for Leo: Onyx, rose quartz, tiger's eye, sunstone, carnelian, garnet

Virgo

Virgo is an earth sign with the Maiden, or Virgin, as a glyph and symbol. Virgo is ruled by Mercury and is a feminine and earth sign. You possess the strengths and qualities of being loyal, kind, generous, selfless, practical, down-to-earth, analytical, and highly grounded. You are reliable and responsible and have a fine balance between intellect and being analytically-minded, and intuition. You are also very sensual and creative, as much as you thrive in intellectual pursuits you still need to express yourself artistically.

Virgos are patient, wise, perceptive and self-aware with strong and developed observational skills. You also make an excellent friend or lover due to your kind and caring nature.

Best gemstones & crystals for Virgo: Carnelian, aventurine, red jasper, kyanite, jade

Libra

Libra is an air sign symbolized by the Scales. Libras are lovers of truth, justice, fairness and equality, and are also perceptive, wise, intuitive, analytical, cooperative, fair-minded, social, diplomatic and gracious. Libra is ruled by Venus and this represents this sign's peace and harmony loving nature. You are massively turned off by injustice, inequality and coldness and seek balance and cooperation in all you do. You are also highly intelligent and perceptive, and may also possess unique musical or artistic talents & gifts. Reading a book or watching an insightful documentary are highly favored activities for you.

You are one of the most social signs of the zodiac, yet you also need sufficient time for solitude and introspection. You have an intuitive mind and can see beyond the surface.

Best gemstones & crystals for Libra: Peridot, jade, tourmaline, lapis lazuli, labradorite

Scorpio

Scorpio is a water sign represented by the Scorpion. Ruled by Pluto, this sign's modern ruler, and Mars; it's ancient one, Scorpios are brave, passionate, resourceful, loyal, and independent. Due to Pluto's influence there is something very transformational and powerful about you- your energy can be quite intense. But you are also a true friend, an attentive and passionate lover, and emotionally deep. You can, however, be distrusting, jealous, possessive, secretive and even violent at times. Highly intuitive, positively sensitive and emotional-natured, Scorpios are one of the most intense signs of the Zodiac.

You may be interested in the occult, supernatural and spirituality. When young you were wise beyond your years and have the potential to be a spiritual healer or shaman, or at the very least develop your intuition to new levels.

Best gemstones & crystals for Scorpio: Aquamarine, rose quartz, rhodochrosite, obsidian, malachite, citrine

Sagittarius

Sagittarius (Sag) is a fire sign represented by the Archer, or Centaur. Ruled by Jupiter, Sag's are wise, fun-loving, optimistic, joyful, perceptive and philosophical. You are extremely loyal and kind to those you love, however can be very loud and tactless. This is due to your fiery and often over-masculinized nature. However, you have **immense** creative spirit and a natural adventurous side to you. Honesty defines you and some of your favorite activities include reading, immersing yourself in creativity, mastering an instrument, exploring nature and travelling.

You are independent but crave and need social connections and interactions. Philosophically speaking, you seek higher wisdom and truths and are often finding new ways to expand your mind and your horizons.

Best gemstones & crystals for Sagittarius: Topaz, turquoise, amethyst

Capricorn

Capricorn is an earth sign ruled by the planet Saturn, and symbolized by the Goat. This is often referred to as the mountain goat, which portrays your nature of climbing the mountain. You are responsible, highly practical and grounded, down-to-earth, and success minded. You strive for success and achievement and like to push yourself to achieve. You are also sensual, self-controlled, disciplined, and lovers of family, tradition and music. There is an element of tradition to you, yet you equally love getting in tune with your inner wild woman or man.

Creativity is a must in your world and you make a wonderful friend, family member and partner. You are a sweet and sensual lover and can uplift those around you with your sage wisdom and advice.

Best gemstones & crystals for Capricorn: Ruby, hematite, obsidian, jade, peridot, azurite, garnet

Aquarius

Aquarius is also known as the "water-bearer" and is an earth sign ruled by Uranus and Saturn. Aquarius is progressive, original, independent, unconventional, eccentric, intellectual and analytical. Aquarius' enjoy humanitarian interests and causes and learning new things, you are primarily mental and often out of tune with deep emotions. It is not that you are unemotional, it is just that you would rather form and develop intellectual connections. You're wise, perceptive and intelligent but can sometimes be aloof and detached. Music, art and the weird, wacky & peculiar interest you.

Aquarius makes excellent teachers, students, writers, researchers, analysts and artists. Anything that makes use of your mind and inner genius is perfect for you.

Best gemstones & crystals for Aquarius: Garnet, aquamarine, amber, yellow jasper

Pisces

Pisces is the 12th sign of the Zodiac, and symbolizes **completion.** Pisces are known as the **old souls** as they are literally the final sign, thus representing completion and wholeness. Pisces is a water sign symbolized by the Fish (two fish), and this in itself portrays Pisces dual nature. Often "swimming in two different directions," Pisces are incredibly spiritual and sensitive, yet also capable of great success in the physical world. This is due to their visionary and inspirational qualities and aspects. You are imaginative, creative, intuitive, sensitive, spiritually aware, artistic and compassionate. Pisces have a strong sense of idealism, morality and unconditional love- more so than any other sign. You make an incredible artist, musician, seer, prophet, shaman, healer, therapist, astrologer, psychic, visionary, counsellor, social or support worker, carer, or metaphysical teacher.

Pisces is ruled by Neptune, the planet of dreams, the arts, creativity and spirituality. Your ancient ruler is Jupiter, representing expansion, higher consciousness, universal wisdom or truth, and higher ideals. Pisces is the most empathic, intuitive, gifted and soulful sign of the Zodiac. You also encompass the qualities and strengths of all 12 signs! (Hence being called the old souls…)

Conclusion

Throughout history man has used the power of crystals. Most ancient cultures have held crystals as sacred objects and have used them in ceremony, for meditation, to clarify thoughts and to help with healing. Today crystals are integrated into our modern technologies, they are used in communications, computers, medical and laser technologies, yet they retain their appeal as magical talismans.

They are naturally formed by geological processes and are located all over the world in a diverse range of environments. The crystals you see today grew from minerals subjected to intense heat and pressure millions of years ago or as a result of sedimentary action over millennia.

Most of the crystals you know about today came from the earth; however some have arrived here from the heavens or space.

These are known as tektites and meteorites.

www.ingramcontent.com/pod-product-compliance
Lightning Source LLC
Chambersburg PA
CBHW071832080526
44589CB00012B/993